Don't Sweep It Under the Drug!

Don't Sweep It Under the Drug!

INTEGRATING EVIDENCE-BASED BODY MIND & SPIRITUAL PRACTICES INTO YOUR HEALTH & WELLNESS TOOL KIT

Cathy Rosenbaum

Copyright © 2015 Cathy Rosenbaum
All rights reserved.

ISBN 13: 9781512368123
ISBN 10: 1512368121
Library of Congress Control Number: 2015908462
CreateSpace Independent Publishing Platform
North Charleston, South Carolina

Disclaimer

This book is not meant to take the place of personal advice from your doctor, pharmacist, or other healthcare professional. Do not act upon any information without consulting a doctor who knows your medical, surgical, prescription-drug, over-the-counter drug, and dietary-supplement history. This book is intended only to help educate you and provide information for discussion with your doctor.

Reference to any former clients is purely coincidental. All of the individual consultation scenarios presented in this book are fictitious. Conditions from more than one client have been combined for the sake of illustration. Names have been changed.

Dedication

To the Lord, who gave me talents and a calling to serve others. To my father and mother, who raised me with Christian values and a desire to pursue goodness, stewardship, a thirst for nature, music, and a strong work ethic. To my sons, daughters-in-law, and grandchildren, who have kept me anchored in the value of paying it forward with unconditional love.

Table of Contents

Chapter 1 Introduction ··· 1

Chapter 2 My Unexpected Calling into Integrative
and Holistic Health and Medicine ···························· 6

Chapter 3 The Prescription-Drug Industry:
Who Moved the FDA's Cheese? ···························· 14

Chapter 4 Herbs, Other Dietary Supplements, and Nutrition:
Dance Partners or Double-Edged Swords? ·················· 27

Chapter 5 Complementary and Alternative Medicine:
A Brave New World ··· 36

Chapter 6 Personalized Health and Wellness:
The Eight-Balance-Point Model for Healing ················ 43

Chapter 7 Combating Superstress with Guided Imagery ············· 56

Chapter 8 Aromatherapy: Lavender's Blue (Dilly, Dilly) ············· 61

Chapter 9 Spiritual Renewal: Exploring Life's Mysteries ············· 64

CHAPTER 1

Introduction

> *In all affairs it's a healthy thing to hang a question mark on the things you have long taken for granted.*
> —BERTRAND RUSSELL

Remember Ernestine, Lily Tomlin's telephone operator from TV's *Laugh-In*? Just like her trademark "One ringy dingy, two ringy dingies," I'm calling y'all, boomers. Have I reached the party to whom I am speaking? By now, most of us have figured out that health, delight, wisdom, and a sense of purpose are not solely dependent on the condition of our bodies as portrayed in the media. Certainly, our life journey can be more pleasant when our physical health is optimal, but maintaining physical health alone often comes at the cost of being out of tune with other aspects of life. While "rebalancing an imbalanced life" is in vogue, I am guessing few of us routinely focus on our emotional and spiritual health as much as on our physical health and appearance. It's no wonder—we live in a country obsessed with age avoidance. Commercials on television encourage us to buy products to remove wrinkles, cover age spots, and stay youthful as long as possible. This sounds like plain avoidance. Remember what Phyllis Diller told us: "Old age is when the liver spots show through your gloves." My response? Wear heavier gloves. Good-bye to the unsolicited AARP card, and hello to Phyllis's shot of wisdom about wearing apparel. The body is a holy temple for our mind and spirit. We should be good stewards of each aspect of it. Phyllis also told us, "Housework can't kill you, but why take a chance?" What did she know? There is no time better than the present for some lifestyle and medicine-cabinet housecleaning.

This book is titled *Don't Sweep It Under the Drug!* The first question to answer is, what is "it"? The answer is, "your life journey." Like many of you, I grew up in the 1960s, a turbulent time in America. Ironically, young people were engaged in revolutionary efforts to find peace and love during postwar chaos. I found one but not the other, and I'll let you guess which one. Do you remember paisley fabric, slide rules, fishnet stockings, exotic earrings, miniskirts, and music from Woodstock? Through high school and my early years in college, I somehow grew up, found my way, and acquired a responsible and fairly healthy lifestyle. I would be interested to know how many of us are leading emotionally, spiritually, and physically balanced lives today.

An important first step toward "booming changes" is to admit we *need* to change. If your earthly journey is complex, fast paced, distressed, overscheduled, full of text messaging, nature deprived, or, in short, excessively out of tune, and you feel like you are missing something, you have found the right book. It's time to learn how to de-stress and face head on some of your emotional and spiritual extra weight. Chronic stress cannot be eliminated entirely, but we baby boomers can certainly take baby steps to minimize the negative effects it has on our health.

Are you wondering where to start? Here are some suggestions: Minimize your use of technology—cell phones and computers. Get back outside to play. And, with direction from your doctor, curb your use of any medications—prescription and over-the-counter—that could be affecting your mind and body negatively.

As a business owner, I see the value in technology that brings us closer to our clients, to the world, and to the latest medical research. But what has technology done to our social interactions, relationship building, and deeper sense of commitment to our communities?

As a pharmacist, I appreciate the use of prescription medications as part of healing interventions, such as antibiotics for bacterial infections, medications for heart arrhythmias, and insulin for diabetes mellitus. Let's face it: we're getting to an age when taking medications can be as routine as brushing our teeth. I'm gently pushing against the ethical pharmaceutical-industry machine, or Pharmaceutical Research and Manufacturers of America (PhRMA), because of concern over long-term medication side effects. I'm guessing you feel the same way, and that is why you are reading this book. You will be illuminated on how to handle aging in a healthy way without resorting to an abundance of prescription medications and dietary supplements.

Who among my fellow healthcare professionals is out there promoting simpler lifestyles and educating the public about evidence-based, nonmedication-related interventions for health? The book is a call to action. It is not intended to convince readers to sell their laptops, discontinue their high-speed Internet services, go live in the wilderness without indoor plumbing, talk for hours to strangers about pet hobbies, or completely stop taking prescription medications. Rather, this book will help you think about ways to simplify your whole life—to relax and seek out the basics of living.

The book is also not an encyclopedia of herbal and alternative remedies used to replace prescription medications for various chronic conditions. If you bought it for that reason, I appreciate the donation to the greater cause of health. However, you will quickly find out that I do not make generalized recommendations to dear souls unless I know their complete health history. Please note that the names of clients portrayed in this book have been changed to protect their privacy.

Let us begin by creating a list of your body, mind, and spiritual blessings. They could include a house, food on the table, family, friends, freedom to worship, or a job. Write down these blessings, and then set them aside. We'll come back to them in chapter 6.

A car requires preventive maintenance to keep it in good running condition, so we periodically have it serviced. Belts, hoses, fluids, and brakes get poked and pulled. If we put off repairs too long, the cost to restore the car to good working order is much higher. Similarly, there comes a time in our own lives when we need a fifty-thousand-mile health tune-up. Many of us take better care of our cars than ourselves. We have collected a lot of dirt over the years, and it's time for a good dusting and cleaning of our mind, body and spirit as well as our medicine and dietary supplement chests. These two notions go hand in hand.

If you have reached age fifty, you have lived nearly 438,000 hours. Approximately 109,000 of those hours have been used for sleep when you get an average of six hours per night. How many of those hours have been spent in deep, restorative rapid-eye-movement (REM) sleep, when we experience healing? Did you know that lack of sleep can affect your eating habits as well as overall health?

Some of us take a casual approach to our personal health. As the sayings go, "If it ain't broke, don't fix it," and "Parts is parts." Perhaps we don't feel the need for preventive measures, or we may not be ready to change, or we are too busy caring for others to think about it. Remember the old saying "An ounce of prevention is worth a pound of cure"? After so many laps around life's racetrack, we need body, mind, and spiritual adjustments. Putting off important maintenance, including time to refuel, can lead to chronic illness. How can we get back on track? These chapters will provide ideas to build your own tool kit of health tips. Share them with your doctor and other evidence-based, nontraditional medicine practitioners in your community who care about you as a whole person.

Seventy-eight million Americans were born in the post–World War II era, from 1946 through 1964. I'm one of them. Every day through 2029, approximately ten thousand baby boomers in America will reach sixty-five years of age, according to AARP data. Our generation has worked hard, fought for causes we believe in, and sought equal partnership on our health team. Many of us believe healthcare with lots of options and freedom of choice is our right in a time when choices seem to be narrowing within the context of the Affordable Care Act. (Now, don't drag me into politics, because I will not go there. It's not politically correct in a book about healing—too stressful). Whether you work inside or outside of your home or have retired, this book can better inform you on how to make whole-person health choices.

The book will encourage you to unmask your inner emotions, draw closer to your spiritual self, keep your physical engine in optimal working order, and see the big picture of accountability to your family and community in a way that ultimately contributes to your *own* inner peace. You will learn more about specific nontraditional health and medicine practices others have tried with success. You might want to further explore these methods with the guidance of your doctor or your integrative and holistic clinical pharmacist.

What's the point to all this work? It is my hope that you will learn more about my whole-person, back-to-basics approach to living and be drawn to a desire to serve others. Get ready to reinvent yourself and talk with your doctor about developing a healthcare team to accomplish your goals. Think of this effort as a fun adventure. Pretend it is sweeps week at your house and your health-journey ratings are about to go up. Gentlemen and ladies, start your engines (oops, I mean electric brooms). Good luck!

CHAPTER 2
My Unexpected Calling into Integrative and Holistic Health and Medicine

> *Go forth into the busy world and love it. Interest yourself in its life, mingle kindly with its joys and sorrows.*
> —Ralph Waldo Emerson

Perhaps the Byrds sang it best in their 1960s song "Turn! Turn! Turn!": "There is a season…and a time for every purpose under heaven." Bible readers may recall this passage from Ecclesiastes 3:1. When I was sixteen, I decided I wanted to become a pharmacist, even though I had not taken any chemistry classes or explored other options. Most of my college education was quite fulfilling and routine. I went the traditional route of getting a bachelor's degree, which was followed by a doctorate in pharmacy ten years later. I practiced mostly in hospitals, taught pharmacy students, and became involved in medical affairs and safety surveillance within industry. In 2000 I went back to school and got an MBA. The summer after my graduation, I was sitting in a lounge chair in the middle of my driveway when I looked to the sky and asked, "What is next, Lord?" Little did I know that my professional life was about to change. It began with an exciting job as an administrator for an integrative health and medicine center.

But there is more to the story. Beyond the births of my two children, I have had many significant experiences that one could term miracles. These were miracles of healing. They began after my father's diagnosis with a rare type of cancer, a serendipitous trip to China, and my father's subsequent passing into heaven.

There are only two ways to live your life:
One is as though nothing is a miracle.
The other is as if everything is.
I believe in the latter.

—ALBERT EINSTEIN

Who would have guessed Einstein felt that way? Do you believe in miracles? When I was growing up, I thought miracles were given to a select few mentioned in the Bible, but not to me or anyone close. The healing of the blind man, the raising of Lazarus from the dead—these familiar stories seemed more like dreams than reality. Yet when our loved ones become gravely ill, we oftentimes pray for miraculous healings even though we seldom expect to see them. Should we not believe?

What I am about to tell you may change your mind. The story is an awesome example of several incredible experiences, and it begins with my dad. In 1997, Dad received his first diagnosis of cancer. For the next several years, he underwent multiple surgeries, chemotherapy, and radiation. He passed away in 2006, within twenty-four hours of the passing of his only brother, in the same town, of unrelated causes. How often does that happen in life? Dad's story of "nine lives" explains how God got my attention.

The son of German farmers, Dad was a bright and talented child. He and his brother were asked to work in their father's lumber mill at a young age. The brothers were very close and looked out for each other. Dad saw a lot in his life growing up as he lived through the Depression and World War II. For three years he fought in the army on the front line, in the European theater under General George Patton, but he was not physically harmed. That was the first miracle, even though we are sure there were emotional scars from what he saw and had to do to protect our country. After the war, Dad went on to become a mechanical engineer, with only two years of college. He had to work to help support the family. Dad instilled in me a strong work ethic and an eye for quality.

To say I feared my father would be an understatement. He expected perfection in himself and everyone around him. During my teenage years, my fear turned into typical childhood discontent. Dad was a formidable force in my life but always maintained high Christian values in our home.

Years later, I would be able to find similarities in my compassion for his childhood suffering and the anguish he bore in his final months on earth.

One day in 1997, I received a phone call from my mother telling me about Dad's cancer, a sarcoma in his leg. The biopsy showed that the cancer was at a very advanced stage. The doctors had to make a decision quickly whether or not to operate. My eldest son, my mother, and I walked slowly and methodically into the doctor's office with Dad. Would Dad have to lose his leg and a part of his pelvis, or could the leg be saved with this surgery? We were all frozen with fear. My father's case was recommended to a specialized surgeon in our small town. This surgeon was able to remove the tumor and save Dad's leg. Miracle number two. After the surgery, my son, who was age twenty at the time, spent a week at Dad's side in the hospital and encouraged his grandpa to get well. Today, that son is a physician.

Later, a postoperative histologic test indicated that Dad's tumor had spread up the sciatic nerve, but the local pathologist was unsure of the findings because the tumor was so uncommon. The tissue sample was sent to the Mayo Clinic for a second opinion. Two long weeks later, we were told there was no metastasis after all. After Dad underwent several rounds of intense radiation, his cancer was considered to be in remission. That first cancer never returned. Miracle number three.

During the year after this first surgery, doctors discovered that Dad had an abdominal aortic aneurysm needing urgent repair. He had more surgery, and again it was successful. But there were problems with his blood pressure through the night related to some of the medications used in the operating room. My mother and I were standing watch at the hospital that night, shoring each other up. Mother broke down several times from fear and exhaustion. Many thoughts and emotions flooded my mind. "Did I tell Dad I loved him? Did he know how much we needed him?" After four agonizing hours, we were told he was OK.

As Dad recovered at home, I would sit and rub his feet to distract him and ease the pain from his surgical wounds, not knowing what else to do for him. I wanted to comfort him and express my love in a tangible way as he had been through so much. Touch is one of the five languages of love. Our relationship blossomed through those days and weeks, and my ability to express love for him in a different way was made very real. This was the fourth miracle.

During one of two additional major surgeries for unrelated issues in the months ahead, Dad had an unexpected reaction to a medication used to prevent infection, coded, was revived, and later was placed in the ICU. He survived this event, too. This was miracle number five.

Months after his last surgery, Dad developed chronic lymphocytic leukemia, which the doctors thought was caused by the radiation used to treat his sarcoma. By this time, our family came to believe that Dad could defy the odds. We began to expect another miracle, not to be surprised by one.

More time passed after the diagnosis of his second cancer, and Dad became acutely sick again. The doctors saw shadows in his lungs and feared the worst—could it be metastatic cancer? It turned out that Dad's appendix had ruptured and abscessed. His appendix was removed, the abscess was drained, and he survived. Miracle number six. While he was recovering in the ICU, I would sit and watch him breathe and sleep quietly. I would put a cool cloth on his forehead to soothe him even though he was heavily sedated.

The first few weeks before and after Dad's first surgery and the years thereafter were emotionally and spiritually challenging and caused me to question God. Many times, I wondered whether I could trust that God would spare Dad's life for us to be able to witness our love for him, and for God, in a way that we had never been able to do before.

Just after Dad's five-year anniversary for sarcoma remission, the leukemia returned. Dad received beginning rounds of more chemotherapy, was given a medication to prevent blood clots, and bled unexpectedly from his colon. The entire supply of his blood type in the hospital's blood bank had nearly been exhausted, and surgery was again necessary to save his life. Dad came through it just fine. This was miracle number seven.

Two weeks before Dad died, I woke up one night with a horrible feeling. I began to pace the floor and cry out, "Daddy, Daddy!" I was so distraught that I fell down a flight of stairs, but I did not get severely hurt. This was a sign from above. Miracle number eight. God appeared to be preparing me for the transition. During the fourth of five rounds of chemotherapy, right before Thanksgiving, Dad died peacefully in his sleep. Nine long years had passed. That he died near a significant wedding anniversary, at a holiday time when his family could be together, and that he could leave in peace with his brother after all this suffering was miracle number nine. He fought long and hard.

Now, have you changed your mind about miracles? I have been forever changed. God used Dad's journey to bless me with a renewed desire to help others in need. Why did all those miracles take place? In *The Heart of a God Chaser*, Tommy Tenney says "chasers" have hunger that exceeds their reach. Why do miracles happen to some and not others? Could it be because some are hungrier to see them than others? In *Small Miracles—Extraordinary Coincidences from Everyday Life*, Yitta Halberstam and Judith Leventhal give us examples of countless coincidences, the seemingly random acts that turn out not to be so random at all. They are remarkable happenings, wonderful examples of God working in our lives. My dad's illness and his incredible journey showed me so much about love and healing. Those experiences began to change me professionally before I realized it. I was too busy watching his miracles unfold.

If you want to chase miracles in your own life, start by keeping a journal and watching the world through your spiritual eyes. Listen to that still voice inside you. Write about your emotions and how you may react to situations involving the deep mysteries of life. Then spiritually reflect on what you have seen and on the message these events have for you.

For those struggling with a loss, I offer a poem by Iris Bolton to help ease your pain. Start each day expecting ordinary miracles in your life.

I don't know why...
I'll never know why...
I don't like it...
I don't have to like it...

What I do have to do is make a choice about my living.
What I do have to do is accept it and go on living.
The choice is mine.

I can go on living, valuing every moment in a way I never did before, or I can be destroyed by it and, in turn, destroy others.

I thought I was immortal, that my children and my family were also, that tragedy happened only to others.
But I know now that life is tenuous and valuable.

And I choose to go on living, making the most of the time I have, and valuing my family and friends in a way I never did before.

Let us go back to the time of my professional epiphany on a happier note. In the middle of Dad's illnesses, I woke up one morning after completing my MBA program and felt an overwhelming calling to start a service-oriented business, but I was unsure of all the details. Later, I realized it was the Holy Spirit nudging me in that particular direction. Another miracle came my way in 2002. I was invited to travel to China with a professional group from People to People International. We visited Beijing and Chengdu to study herbal and pharmaceutical drug research, comparing regulatory requirements of the US Food and Drug Administration (FDA) to those of the State Food and Drug Administration of China (SFDA). Our group was made up of medical doctors, doctors of pharmacy, and PhD biochemists from around the United States. During the trip we interacted with the Chinese government, representatives from the pharmaceutical industry, and colleagues from the Chengdu University of Traditional Chinese Medicine. At the university we saw rooms full of natural herbs and medicinals separated into animal, vegetable, and mineral categories. We talked with colleagues at a barefoot doctor clinic in Chengdu in Sichuan province in southwestern China. Historically, these doctors were first farmers. The name "barefoot" traditionally came from southern farmers who worked barefoot in their rice paddies and then went on to receive minimal medical training to be able to work in rural clinics where traditional doctors would not go. The doctors we met were wearing shoes. We saw a dirty, primitive operating room, a delivery room, a room devoted to cardiac patients, and areas for massage and acupuncture treatments. There was a small, rustic, one-room pharmacy on site with raw herbs collected in wooden vats. The barefoot doctor would scoop up combinations of these herbs, brew them into a tea, place the tea in a large container, and serve it to the patients. We were told those teas smelled and tasted awful, but they seemed to help comfort and heal many of the patients, according to the doctor. Teas were customized to each patient's needs. In that pharmacy, we also saw modern medications such as boxes of Abbott's dextrose 5 percent in water for intravenous infusions.

Next, we traveled to Beijing to witness government-sponsored pharmaceutical research in a modern, high-technology hospital. We spoke with government officials, representatives of the pharmaceutical industry, and Chinese academicians. Several of us gave presentations on our professional research topics of interest. We discussed how prescription medication research was being conducted in the United States and what the FDA required of it compared with the SFDA process in China. We compared the rigor of pharmaceutical research to the typical lack thereof regarding herbs and other dietary supplements worldwide. We toured the Beijing Institute of Genomics and the Chinese Academy of Sciences and learned about a rice-modification project and the human genome project.

The group observed through our Chinese colleagues' eyes an understanding that there is so much more to the human experience of healing than the physical aspect. Digging even deeper, an intriguingly different path to health starts with a back-to-basics lifestyle coupled with respect for the elderly and community respect and responsibility—concepts I found halfway around the world and wanted to bring back to America. This integrative health model has come to the United States and is gaining momentum thirteen years later. The enhanced model combines Eastern and Western medical principles and places equal emphasis on psychosocial, spiritual, and physical healing interventions.

After the China trip, I was forever changed and immediately started a consulting practice helping others learn more about dietary supplements, how they work, the evidence—or lack thereof—behind their indications, and how to find quality products. Early on, I simply wondered about the evidence behind mind-body-spiritual healing, having experienced some of it with Eastern practitioners. Today, I have expanded these consultations to include discussion and tips for emotional and spiritual healing while deemphasizing medications and supplements and promoting the less complicated lifestyle choices that many baby boomers crave. I still work at a local hospital in medication quality and safety. I ultimately want to help bridge the gap between doctors and evidence-based nontraditional health and medicine practitioners, share with each of them the comprehensive whole-person model for healing that I saw in China, and help build a healthcare team with patients as equal partners in the decision-making process.

I hope these life stories help you better understand why I am trying to inspire a change in the landscape of medical intervention from prescription medications first and only, to more conservative prescribing in which medications are used last in the list of options for healing whenever possible. From time spent in the pharmaceutical industry, I have learned that medications are important in treatment and the industry is not all bad. To discover how our country has become enamored with dietary supplements, we first have to understand more about concerns regarding long-term use of medications. You will find out why in the next chapter.

CHAPTER 3

The Prescription-Drug Industry: Who Moved the FDA's Cheese?

> *A miracle drug is any drug that will do what the label says it will do.*
> —Eric Hodgins

Mirror, mirror on the wall, who is the fairest perimenopausal maiden of them all? More like a damsel in distress, you say. Sally is a fifty-something-year-young baby boomer referred to me by her ob-gyn for a consultation on hormone-replacement-therapy alternatives to help her handle her unwanted symptoms of menopause. Are there any *wanted* symptoms? It's not like we stand in line signing up for hot flashes, mood swings, and other symptoms that go bump in the night. Most of the time, women will associate these changes with dramatic estrogen fluctuations over several years and oftentimes manage them with prescription hormone-replacement therapy. Other times, suppressed emotional issues such as anxiety or depression that have been with them for life are unmasked. Regardless of the cause, challenging symptoms are knocking at the door and must be greeted with multiple types of healing interventions. Who is the hospitality chairperson, and where is the dust mop? We have some more housework to do.

Very few women get through their menopausal years without some kind of prescription or over-the-counter pharmaceutical intervention. Sally and I discussed the pros and cons of prescription-hormone therapy, bioidentical compounded prescription hormones, phytoestrogen herbal supplements, phytoestrogenic foods, and much more related to emotional and spiritual healing. Her goal was to maintain physical strength and vitality. It's important to note that Sally has a history of fibrocystic breast disease, which can make breast-cancer detection by routine mammogram more difficult. Sally received soy formula as an infant, took birth control pills in her early marriage, ate lots of hormone-fed chicken, started taking black cohosh for her menopausal hot flashes, and knew that her hubby sprayed their lawn with pesticides containing xenoestrogens every spring. Her mother died of breast cancer when she was in her sixties.

Sally chose to stay away from prescription hormones because of concerns about the risk of breast cancer associated with continuous use. Together, we developed a tool kit of nonmedication interventions to help manage her bone and heart health mainly through exercise, stress management, and whole-food nutrition. Sally has done well through her postmenopausal years. She has learned to play a musical instrument and has gone through her transition with grace. She is managing her emotional heart, as well as her physical heart, with style. Let us applaud Sally for handling menopause without hormone-replacement therapy. Unfortunately, Sally's story is not representative of the majority of women I see.

Why do Americans take so many medications? We have seen the "direct-to-consumer" TV commercials for drugs encouraging us to talk with our doctors about the newest products on the market. According to these ads, savvy patients should expect any and all of these medications to be prescribed immediately by their caring doctors. As a result we oftentimes end up taking more medications to treat the side effects resulting from the first medication prescribed, and so on. It is a vicious cycle. I have seen patients taking ten to fifteen medications multiple times each day (and even more dietary supplements) because of efficient advertising and medication savings cards given by the drug companies. "Direct-to-professional" advertising is more health- and cost-efficient.

According to the 2012 IMS Institute for Healthcare Informatics Report, per-capita retail-prescription usage averaged 11.33 medications per person, placing many patients at risk of unwanted drug interactions and side effects. Nearly fifty million people ages fifty-seven to eighty-five are estimated to regularly take at least one prescription drug (Qato 2008). When doctors change prescriptions, modify a dose, or add more prescriptions to the treatment regimen, the burden of medication education for the consumer increases dramatically. Oftentimes, medication adherence becomes more difficult. For those who must take prescription drugs for chronic health conditions, it may not be too late to make some positive changes and reduce the need to continue some of them. For many it is possible to either decrease the medication dose or eliminate the need to take a particular medication altogether if less invasive lifestyle interventions are made and maintained. It takes some coordination with your medical doctor, an ounce of discipline, time, and a belief that lifestyle simplification can make a difference. If this approach is successful, you will experience a reduced risk of medication errors and side effects.

Let us talk about the Food and Drug Administration (FDA) and how ethical prescription drugs are regulated in the US market. Before we can talk about nontraditional health and medicine and healing with minimal use of prescription medications, we need to respect the laws governing the ethical drug-development process. The FDA is responsible for enforcing laws enacted by Congress. Stephen Ostroff, MD, is the acting FDA commissioner. Get to know more about him professionally and about his job responsibilities. The FDA is one of the strictest regulatory agencies in the world, but we need it. Congress has enacted laws outlining the procedures a manufacturer must follow to obtain marketing approval of a drug. The FDA faces unparalleled challenges when it comes to monitoring drug quality and safety because of pressure from the ethical pharmaceutical industry (PhRMA). PhRMA spends billions of dollars on lobbying Congress, and our government, in turn, does not set limits on drug price increases as other countries do. Drug prices in the United States rose 8 percent a year from 2006 through 2011. The rate at which prescription-drug costs increased between 2014 and 2015 was 13 percent. This rate was driven by the introduction of new specialty drugs, an increase in compound drugs, and price increases for both brand-name and generic drugs. High drug prices, in turn, affect health-insurance premiums and the Medicare bucket. PhRMA does not allow Medicare to negotiate prices with drug manufacturers. The system is far from perfect and needs repair. It will take more than a dust mop or a bucket and rag to clean up that mess.

Overuse of prescription medications has created problems in the United States. Narcotics often are prescribed for pain management, and use of the products carries the risk of fatal overdoses. To avoid getting narcotics into the hands of the wrong people, such as children, other family members, or potential medication abusers, be sure to discard any unused medications once you are finished with them, and do not save or share them. Disposal options include flushing the drugs down the toilet, using medication take-back programs administered through local authorities or collectors authorized by the Drug Enforcement Administration (DEA), or mixing unwanted or leftover crushed narcotic medications with coffee grounds or cat litter before disposing of them in household trash.

Solving the complex problems involving medication overuse requires the efforts of healthcare professionals and consumers alike. For more information on interventional assistance to manage prescription-drug addiction, visit http://www.stopyouraddiction.com/addiction-treatment-faqs/what-do-family-members-need-to-know-about-drug-abuse-treatment.

Back to the FDA. Here is how it works: Over-the-counter- (OTC) and prescription-medication research is regulated by an FDA branch called the Center for Drug Evaluation and Research (CDER). To market a new drug in the United States, the sponsor first must demonstrate positive results in test tubes and animal preclinical studies to gather efficacy, toxicity, and pharmacokinetic data. Next are the human studies.

The first phase of human study uses normal volunteers to explore dose-ranging with subtherapeutic as well as ascending doses. Studies during this phase focus mostly on drug safety and involve twenty to one hundred people to determine whether the drug can have efficacy.

Studies in the second phase are the first controlled trials in one hundred to three hundred patients that examine the preliminary effectiveness and safety of a therapeutic drug dosage. Does the product do what it is supposed to do if taken according to directions?

Phase-three studies are expanded, randomized, double-blind, controlled trials in one thousand to two thousand patients. Their focus is on the drug's effectiveness, efficacy, and safety. These studies are used to evaluate the overall benefit-to-risk relationship of the drug. At this stage of research, the drug is administered in its anticipated commercial strength or dosage. Studies conducted in this phase may involve comparison of the proposed product with available prescription drugs used for the same indication or to a placebo control arm. Results from these trials are used to supply more information to healthcare professionals for clinical decision making. Finally, phase-four (or postmarketing surveillance) studies are conducted after the drug is FDA approved for marketing to monitor how the product is actually used by millions of people in the real-world setting (e.g., as it is intended or otherwise). Phase-four studies are typically focused on product safety.

A control group is important in a clinical research study to remove bias. A placebo, or sugar pill, does not contain any active drug ingredients. A study is called double-blind when neither the study participant nor the research investigator knows whether the drug or placebo is being administered, because they look identical. To receive FDA approval to market the drug in the United States, only two double-blind, randomized, placebo-controlled clinical studies are required from the drug manufacturer. Are you surprised? It's important to note that short-term, company-sponsored clinical research cannot determine all of a drug's long-term (ten to twenty years) side effects in the general population, whose use may be different from those in the studies.

The FDA reviews hundreds of drug trials a year. Healthcare professionals use other published medical information to monitor the safety and efficacy of prescription drugs, including case reports, cohort studies, meta-analyses, and epidemiological studies. Drug registries, poison-control-center reports, and drug-manufacturer-generated phase-four postmarketing surveillance safety reports are other ways consumers can find out about a drug's safety profile.

To protect the consumer, a drug manufacturer must follow current Good Manufacturing Practices (cGMP). This means that all processes pertaining to a drug's production must maintain product identity, dose strength, product quality, and purity.

To make matters even more challenging, there is a shortage of prescription medications in the United States. Managing this shortage requires a team of creative healthcare professionals across this country to keep up with the changing drug-supply chain. The number of new drug shortages per year rose from 130 in 2007 to nearly 267 through 2011 and continues to be well over one hundred each year thereafter. Shortages include generic sterile injectable products, anticancer drugs, anesthetic agents, pain medications, and nutritionals, creating an estimated annual effect on US hospitals of $216 million from the purchase of medication alternatives.

"Why does this happen?" you ask. Multiple factors contribute to drug shortages. Here are a few examples:

- Raw material shortages. Nearly 80 percent of pharmaceutical-grade raw materials are sourced outside of the United States. Drug availability can be affected when political instability interrupts trade with foreign countries, animal diseases contaminate tissue from which raw materials are harvested, or environmental issues affect plant growth from which raw materials are sourced. The drug heparin was recalled in March 2008 as a result of Chinese adulteration of injectable heparin with oversulfated chondroitin. Heparin is an anticoagulant used for the treatment of clots in deep leg veins and lungs.
- Quality issues. Nearly 42 percent of sterile injectable-drug shortages in 2010 were caused by product-quality issues, such as particulates, microbial contamination, or stability changes.
- Manufacturing difficulties or production decisions. Business decisions regarding branded drugs are made every day based on availability of generic drugs, the product's market size, patent expirations, drug-approval status, and anticipated clinical demand for the product. Manufacturers are not required to report product discontinuations to the FDA unless they are the sole source of a life-supporting medication or a medication used to prevent a debilitating disease. Occasionally, consumer loyalty to branded products decays with the advent of newer products within the same drug class. Over time there is a diminishing financial return on a brand to the manufacturer, and the company will remove that branded product from its portfolio.
- Change in product formulation. Product-line extensions and formulation changes can evolve for marketing reasons, safety reasons, or both. In 2006 there was a transition from albuterol and other metered-dose inhalers with chlorofluorocarbons for people with chronic obstructive pulmonary disease (COPD) to metered-dose inhalers containing hydrofluoroalkanes, which are safer alternatives.
- Regulatory issues. As stated earlier in this chapter, the FDA enforces drug-manufacturing standards called current Good Manufacturing

Practices (cGMP). The FDA also helps manufacturers that are not in cGMP compliance return to compliance when a significant corrective action involves a medically necessary product. But the FDA does not have the authority to require a manufacturer to produce any drug, even if the drug is a medical necessity.

- Industry consolidation and company mergers. Mergers frequently involve closing manufacturing facilities and narrowing the drug-product portfolios of the postmerger corporations.
- Restricted drug distribution and allocation. A drug manufacturer can place restrictions on limited drug supplies by requiring that its drug be sourced through a specialty distributor.
- Just-in-time inventory (JIT). JIT is a strategy to minimize costs at various points along the drug-supply chain. Some drug shortages may be dependent on wholesalers, as drug shortages can occur when contracts with suppliers are delayed. The wholesaler charges the manufacturers for stocking their drugs, and the manufacturers restrict the wholesalers from overstocking.
- Changes in product demand and shifts in clinical practice. When a new indication for a marketed drug is FDA approved, when prescribers start ordering the drug for hospital programs (approving the drug for hospital formulary), or when a drug representative promotes new drug products to office- and hospital-based prescribers, generating unanticipated demand, it may be more difficult for pharmacies to keep up with drug-product supply.
- Gray market. The number of licensed "gray" distributors that buy directly from the manufacturers to stockpile scarce drugs and resell at much higher prices is increasing as shortages continue. Purchasing from the gray market does not ensure drug pedigree, especially if the drug is sourced outside of the United States. Drug pedigree is law in Florida and other states where most of the gray market wholesalers are located, but it is not law in Ohio, where I practice.
- Natural disasters. If a fire, earthquake, or tornado struck one manufacturing plant, the company would have to decrease production of one drug at a different plant to continue producing a critical, lifesaving drug at the involved plant.

Some drug-shortage issues are improving. In Febuary 2011 Senator Amy Klobuchar (D-MN) and representative Diana DeGette (D-CO) introduced bipartisan legislation (SB 296 and HR 2245) requiring drug manufacturers to notify the FDA at least six months in advance when a planned interruption in a drug's production could result in a shortage, or as soon as possible if an unexpected interruption or adjustment in supply transpires. The bill supported development of contingency plans for drugs vulnerable to shortage, but it was never enacted. This legislation would not have completely eliminated drug-shortage problems in US hospital pharmacies, retail pharmacies, or physicians' offices. On October 31, 2011, President Obama issued an executive order directing the FDA to expand its reporting of prescription drugs and speed up regulatory review to respond to shortages. For more information visit http://www.fda.gov/Drugs/DrugSafety/DrugShortages/ucm050796.htm.

Managing Polypharmacy

Polypharmacy means regularly consuming five or more medications or purchasing medications from multiple pharmacies. Americans consume more prescription medications than people in any other country. In 2002 the General Accounting Office created a report to congressional requesters titled *Prescription Drugs. FDA Oversight of Direct-to-Consumer Advertising Has Limitations*. This report indicated prescription-drug spending had increased 18 percent annually from 1997 through 2001 and was the fastest-growing component of healthcare spending in the United States.

Forces that have increased polypharmacy in the past few years include PhRMA, as well as direct-to-consumer advertising in print and broadcast educating consumers about medical conditions and creating pent-up demand for physicians to prescribe more medications. When more medications are used by more people, rare side effects are apt to appear. Prescription-drug side effects (such as reduced bone density from long-term use of proton-pump inhibitors), drug-drug interactions, drug-supplement interactions (Asztalos 2003), drug-food interactions, drug recalls, and drug removals as a result of side effects (e.g., Vioxx) must be managed continually with input from the doctor and pharmacist.

The time is right for doctors to consider different ways to reduce the need for drugs as well as encourage their patients to try noninvasive, evidence-based, holistic regimens including lifestyle changes, stress management, and good nutrition and exercise programs. The process by which doctors can change the landscape of overprescribing to a more conservative approach could include one or more of the following:

- Drug holidays. Prescription drugs are studied for short periods and are not meant to be taken for years on end. Doctors should reassess the continued need for medication every three to six months. These include proton-pump inhibitors such as Prilosec for acid reflux and bisphosphonates such as Fosamax for osteoporosis.
- Alternate drug regimens. Doctors may wish to consider every-other-day dosing of drugs such as Zocor instead of daily-dosing regimens, prescribing one ingredient versus combination-ingredient products, and prescribing topical products versus oral products to minimize long-term side effects.
- Herbs, vitamins, and other dietary supplements. Whenever possible, doctors could consider evidence-based, short-term options to enhance or replace prescription medications. For example, cholesterol-lowering red yeast rice can be taken instead of statins such as Zocor, black cohosh can be used instead of hormone-replacement therapy to treat menopausal hot flashes, and glucosamine hydrochloride for osteoarthritis joint pain can be used instead of nonsteroidal anti-inflammatory drugs (NSAIDs). It's important to remember that any prescription and OTC product as well as dietary supplement can have side effects that need to be considered with a doctor in a benefit-versus-risk discussion.
- Lifestyle choices and healthy whole-food diet. Even when medications are prescribed for long-term treatments, doctors can encourage healthy lifestyle choices and whole nutrition in addition to medications to enhance healing for those with conditions such as GERD, or gastroesophageal reflux disease. Healthy choices also can include raising the head of the bed for improved sleep, deep breathing for stress management, and getting a massage and acupuncture.

One problem with having so many new drugs available on the market is that people run the risk of consuming more than necessary for sustainable health and quality of life. People older than sixty-five represent 14 percent of the American population and take nearly 30 percent of all prescription medications. Boomers, we need to encourage our doctors and one another to push against this machine.

Twenty-nine innovative prescription drugs were approved by the FDA in 2013 (twenty-eight in Japan and thirty in Europe). One day, I recorded the number of prescription-drug commercials during two hours of television. Eight pitches were made to viewers to talk with their doctors about prescription drugs. Enough patients must be asking for these medications during visits to a physician to justify the cost of heavy marketing by PhRMA.

Many consumers shop for the best prices on their prescription drugs or their dietary supplements, resulting in business with more than one pharmacy chain, grocery store, or health-food store, in addition to the Internet. It is always in your best interest to stay with one pharmacy or at least the same retail chain when purchasing medications and supplements. This practice permits pharmacists to have a complete and accurate record of your prescription drugs, dietary supplements, and health conditions. Pharmacists can review your records and make recommendations on how best to take prescription drugs and dietary supplements together. I have taken this practice one step further and worked with interested traditional-medicine doctors to help patients reduce the need for some of these prescription drugs as long as and as much as possible.

Another good practice involves creating a list of questions about your medications for the doctor to answer during your office visits. Never hesitate to ask your doctor questions about your medications. Do not be shy or feel guilty because your doctor is busy. Here is a short list of questions to ask your doctor before beginning an OTC or prescription drug:

- How long do you anticipate I will need to take this drug?
- What are some of the more important side effects with both short-term and long-term use of this drug?
- Will it interact with any of the other drugs or dietary supplements I am taking?

- Why do I need to take several drugs for my disease or condition?
- Is there a lifestyle change, an alternate dosing strategy, or another schedule I can try to keep the side effects at minimum?
- How does this drug work to improve my condition?
- Is there anything else I can do first that is less invasive than taking this drug to manage my condition?

Examples of Long-Term Prescription-Drug Side Effects to Avoid

Once drugs have been used in hundreds of thousands of people, less-common unwanted effects occur that were not seen when the drug was given to only a small number of patients in clinical studies for a shorter period.

In the beginning months, more typically is known about how a drug works for its intended use than about its long-term safety. Full knowledge of a drug's safety profile requires that it be on the market for many years. Drug manufacturers are required to submit periodic drug-safety reports to the FDA. If the FDA sees a trend, it may require the manufacturer to conduct a postmarketing study focused on a safety concern, to add a black-box warning to the drug's package insert related to the safety concern (specifically to alert healthcare professionals about potentially dangerous side effects), to limit the drug's use to specific conditions in which the benefits outweigh the risks, or to withdraw the drug from the market altogether.

Drugs that are FDA approved as safe may eventually be shown to cause serious side effects with longer-term use. For example, NSAIDs—including Celebrex, Motrin, and Naprosyn—can cause stomach ulcers, kidney damage, stroke, increased blood pressure, and liver damage. For perspective, incidents of serious liver damage linked to NSAIDs rose sixfold from 1995 through 2005 (*Pharmacy Practice News* 2008). Long-term use of selective serotonin reuptake inhibitors (SSRIs)—such as Zoloft and Paxil—may cause bone-density issues, and proton-pump inhibitors for GERD can increase the risk of contracting *Clostridium difficile* infection or pneumonia in patients taking certain antibiotics at the same time. Now that the FDA has approved intravenous acetaminophen (APAP) for hospitalized patients, taking more than four grams of APAP by any route daily for prolonged periods may contribute to APAP-related liver damage. However, drug-related liver damage is harder to diagnose than one would imagine. Clinical pharmacists should be informing consumers about these possible long-term effects so the doctor and the patient can share the risk-to-benefit decision before the pharmacist dispenses the medication.

Doctors cannot predict every side effect patients may experience from a drug either on a short-term or long-term basis. Healthcare professionals do have an obligation to stay up to date on the published clinical literature to ensure they are giving their patients the most accurate information on safety. At a minimum, it is important to read any drug information leaflets supplied by the pharmacy or the FDA with your medication when it is prescribed and dispensed to you.

Drug Interactions

A drug interaction is an altering of the effect of one drug (object drug) in a significant way as a result of the administration of another drug (precipitant drug). There are too many drug-to-drug, drug-to-dietary-supplement, and drug-to-food interactions to include in this book. Consult the Mayo Clinic (Mayoclinic.org), the People's Pharmacy (Peoplespharmacy.com), the Livestrong Foundation (Livestrong.org), or the US National Library of Medicine and National Institutes of Health's PubMed.gov site (Pubmed.gov) for more information.

Drug Adulteration

OTC or prescription drugs are withdrawn from the market occasionally because of product adulteration (Cole 2003). Drug manufacturer and FDA-generated recalls happen routinely in the marketplace (see http://www.fda.gov/safety/recalls/default.htm). Years ago, McNeil recalled certain batches of Tylenol, Motrin, and other over-the-counter products contaminated by a chemical found in wooden shipping pallets, which caused nausea, vomiting, and diarrhea in some consumers.

The next chapter will lead us into a similar background and regulatory discussion about the herbal and other dietary-supplement category. Perhaps we have taken the prescription-drug epidemic and moved it over one notch to the over-the-counter supplement world. Inquiring minds want to know. Hint: Get out your shop vac and hang on for the ride. Another cleaning marathon is about to take place.

> *Reality is a crutch for people who can't cope with drugs.*
> —LILY TOMLIN

CHAPTER 4

Herbs, Other Dietary Supplements, and Nutrition: Dance Partners or Double-Edged Swords?

> *What the eyes perceive in herbs or stones*
> *or trees is not yet a remedy;*
> *the eyes see only the dross.*
> —Paracelsus

Americans are spending billions of dollars each year on dietary supplements. One in four to one in five American adult prescription-drug users report that they also take nonvitamin dietary supplements (Gardiner 2007, Eisenberg 1993). Many supplement users I have met over the years start taking these products without the advice of a physician or pharmacist, even though they say they want more involvement from their healthcare professionals (Braun 2010). I often wonder why people take such risks. The marketing message we hear is that dietary supplements are safe, are better than nutrition in whole food, and can treat medical conditions. These nebulous claims are based on nutrition because they are regulated as food, and manufacturers cannot make claims that these supplements act like drugs.

Harold is a forty-eight-year-young obese professional who came to see me at his wife's encouragement. He presented a list of more than twenty supplements, some with duplicate ingredients. Harold had done his research and could articulate his health strategy to me but confessed a lack of understanding when it came to supplement dosing. His long-term goal was to stay in generally good health. I could tell he was skeptical of my professional philosophy that eating a balanced Mediterranean-like diet of whole foods is better than dosing with supplements. He wanted my opinion on the use of these self-prescribed megadoses of supplements. After a three-hour one-on-one consultation, I recommended that Harold simplify his regimen. He did not need five products containing four times the recommended daily dose of glucosamine sulfate to treat osteoarthritis pain. Months after my consultation with Harold, his doctor diagnosed type 2 diabetes and prescribed an oral medication for his condition. Harold's doctor placed more emphasis on his dietary intake than on his supplements. It was a long time before we made any significant progress to simplify Harold's supplement regimen, but he eventually began to understand that drug interactions with supplements were causing some of his health problems, such as high blood pressure. We considered the possibility that his increase in blood sugar, partially caused by glucosamine, could have contributed to his prediabetes and delayed an accurate diagnosis.

Do you notice how frequently the people in your inner circle are inclined to talk about dietary supplements? My clients typically have well-articulated reasons for their use of supplements but don't know what to look for when shopping for them. A high-quality product is hard to come by, and most individuals I meet have not been educated on what comprises quality. If you are one of these people, I want you to start by cleaning out your supplement cabinet. Look for products that are expired, offer no company contact information, have proprietary ingredients bundled into one dose representing many constituents (proprietary blend), or lack product-safety information on the label. You will need the experience of a healthcare professional to help you customize the right combination of supplements to meet your health goals. This is not a one-size-fits-all approach.

Herbs and other dietary supplements can be found easily at health-food stores, grocery stores, retail pharmacies, gas stations, chiropractic offices, some doctors' offices, and online. In addition, commercially grown or homegrown herbs and their active constituents are used as medicine in the forms of teas, cooking spices, whole foods, herbal butter, herb-infused oils, topical creams, decoctions, tinctures, extracts, and essential oils for topical aromatherapy.

The use of the whole herbal plant with many constituents differs from the use of a single chemical ingredient to manage symptoms. This is why we worry about manufacturers making herbs and supplements into drug-like products—for example, pushing one constituent to higher doses that are not clinically studied. Herbalists who cultivate plants for medicinal use should be appropriately trained. Worldwide, many are registered through the American Herbalists Guild or are members or fellows in the College of Practitioners of Phytotherapy or the National Herbalists Association of Australia. For more information please visit the British Herbal Medicine Association (Bhma.info), the National Institute of Medical Herbalists (Nimh.org.uk), and the American Botanical Council (Herbalgram.org). Let us take a closer look at available herbal formulations.

Herbal teas or infusions are water-based preparations. Infusion is the preferred method for extracting fresh active constituents from leafy herbs such as chamomile and peppermint. The key plant part to make tea is typically the leaf or flower. Infusions work well when the active constituents are water soluble. In general (but not always), one cup of hot water is poured over one to two teaspoonful of a dried herb or one tablespoonful of a fresh herb and steeped for five minutes in a covered pot to retain the volatile oils. Then the mixture is strained, and the tea is consumed.

Herbal decoctions are also water based. Active constituents from herb roots, rhizomes, wood, bark, nuts, and some seeds are extracted through this method. The plant parts with active constituents are chopped or ground and placed in a pot with one cup of cold water, brought to a boil, simmered (covered) for ten minutes, and strained. Then the decoction is consumed.

Herbal tinctures can be made with ethanol, vinegar, glycerin, and occasionally with water as the base solution. Tinctures are made through a process called maceration. Final product labeling is typically expressed as a ratio of one to five. This means five milliliters or roughly one teaspoonful of liquid equals one gram of original dried herbs. The next time you visit a health-food store, find an herbal tincture and read the label to help illustrate this information.

A fluid extract (alcoholic) is a more concentrated form of herbal product than a tincture. Herbal extracts are expressed as a ratio of one to one or one to two. For example, this can mean two milliliters or a little less than one-half teaspoonful of liquid equals one gram of original dried herbs. Extracts are made through a percolation technique and require more of the plant's essential oils than tinctures because of different methods of preparation.

Naturally extracted aromatic oils from plants—essential oils—are used in aromatherapy. Aromatherapy application can include aerial diffusion for environmental fragrance, direct vapor inhalation for respiratory decongestion or expectoration, and external topical application for general massage or therapeutic skin care. Essential oils typically are diluted and must be handled with care for safety reasons. Ingestion of diluted or undiluted essential oils is not recommended without the advice and consent of a qualified physician. Aromatherapy will be covered in more detail in chapter 8.

Dietary supplements contain one or more of the following ingredients: a vitamin; a mineral; an herb or other botanical; an amino acid; a dietary substance used to supplement the diet by increasing the total dietary intake; or a concentrate, metabolite, constituent, extract, or combination of any ingredient described, as defined by the FDA. In 1987, 85 percent of modern medications were derived from plants. Currently, only 15 percent are plant based; the rest are chemically manufactured as proprietary products. Growth in the dietary-supplement category over the past few years has skyrocketed with nearly sixty thousand products available worldwide. Far fewer products are known to have medicinal qualities. Consumers are forced to select from a paucity of high-quality products with medicinal value for their health needs from thousands of other products that are not evidence based and may even be unsafe to consume. About fifteen million American adults could be at risk for interactions between their prescription or OTC drugs and dietary supplements. One of them could be you.

The FDA's Center for Safe Food and Nutrition (CSFAN) branch regulates dietary supplements and does not require that they be proved effective prior to marketing. As such, supplement manufacturers do not have to prove their product's effectiveness or even its potency. Dietary supplements could be subpotent or even contaminated and still be on the shelf ready for you to purchase. The federal government does not set standards for ingredient concentrations or recommend daily doses of herbal products (Gurley 2009).

You may wonder where healthcare professionals go to find supplement manufacturing standards. The *German Commission E Monographs* covers approximately three hundred fifty dietary supplements. The *European Scientific*

Cooperative on Phytotherapy covers a few more. The *US Pharmacopeia* (usp.org) and the *US Pharmacopeia Dietary Supplements Compendium* publish some dietary-supplement standards, but not full clinical indications and dosing on all sixty thousand products available worldwide. If you are interested in more reading, other herbal-product references include the *British Herbal Compendium*, the *American Herbal Pharmacopeia*, the *Encyclopedia of Herbal Medicine*, *Potter's Cyclopaedia of Botanic Drugs*, the *British Herbal Pharmacopoeia*, and the *European Pharmacopoeia*.

For perspective, the Institute of Medicine (IOM) establishes recommended daily intake for vitamins and minerals, which are different types of supplements. Many supplement manufacturers market megadoses of these vitamins with nutrition-based claims that they improve health—not to mention increase the purchase price of the product—making it difficult for consumers to choose the best products for their needs. Researchers have said these megadose supplements give the consumer only more expensive urine and may, in fact, be toxic (Expert Group on Vitamins and Minerals 2003).

Dietary supplements have the potential for interactions with drugs and side effects just like prescription drugs. With the high cost of prescriptions, it is tempting to try to replace medications with dietary supplements, although supplements are not covered by most third-party insurance or Medicare. Consumers may believe that dietary supplements are safer, cheaper, and more effective than prescription drugs. Taking larger doses of dietary supplements may not be safe in the long term (Medical Letter on Drugs and Therapeutics 1984). It can be difficult to verify a supplement-associated side effect yourself. If you have unwanted effects from supplements, consult your pharmacist or doctor.

Look to your primary-care doctor to explain any short-term need for supplements, why nutrition and lifestyle changes cannot be tried first, or why the doctor thinks compliance with recommended lifestyle changes is not realistic or anticipated. All dietary supplements should be used sparingly and only as needed to minimize unwanted effects.

Dietary-Supplement Regulation

In 1994 Congress established the Dietary Supplement Health and Education Act (DSHEA). This act, an amendment to the US Federal Food,

Drug, and Cosmetic Act, created a regulatory framework to address the safety and labeling of dietary supplements. DSHEA actually reduced the authority of the FDA to regulate herbs. Dietary-supplement manufacturers can make vague claims about supporting the body's structure if the label states that the "FDA has not reviewed or approved this product for use as a drug." Herbs and other dietary supplements cannot make direct claims of preventing or treating disease and are regulated as food by the FDA.

The FDA has the burden of proof to show that a supplement possesses a significant risk to the public and must be removed from the market. This happens, but not frequently. Under DSHEA the supplement manufacturer is responsible for seeing to it that the product is *safe* before it is marketed. The FDA can take action against an unsafe dietary supplement only after it is marketed. Dietary-supplement manufacturers can, and often do, make statements that are untrue and may make nutrition-based claims that are misleading.

After a dietary supplement is marketed, the FDA monitors product safety by requiring the manufacturer to voluntarily report supplement-related adverse events. Because this process is voluntary, it is basically ineffective in keeping consumers and healthcare professionals informed. Furthermore, some adverse reactions are not likely to be causally attributed to the dietary supplement because many people think they are safe.

In 1995 President Clinton appointed a commission to review supplement labels and to make changes. As part of a US law that took effect in 1999, facts labels are required on all supplement packages. Still, wide variances have been reported in labeling compared with the actual content or potency of supplemental ingredients. This can include having very little active constituents in the product or having more of the intended actives than is stated on the label. In February 2015, Hagens Berman filed a class-action lawsuit against Walmart, Walgreens, GNC, and Target over claims of fraudulent supplements. Buyer beware. Because many supplements are made from plants, extracting active constituents from plant materials whose medicinal content is variable can be difficult. Frequently, there is no easy way to determine the effectiveness of a dose or even whether it is effective at all.

The term "natural" used to describe herbal products and other dietary supplements does not always mean "safe." A manufacturer's use of the terms "standardized," "verified," or "certified" may not guarantee product quality, either, unless it is a US Pharmacopeia (USP)-verified dietary supplement. Once a dietary supplement is marketed, the FDA monitors product claims and information on the label and package inserts. The Federal Trade Commission regulates product advertising and requires that information be truthful. To stay current on dietary-supplement-related safety issues, visit Dietary Supplement Alerts and Safety Information on the FDA website (fda.gov) or Alerts and Advisories on the National Center for Complementary and Integrative Health's website (nccih.nih.gov).

Consumer Labs (ConsumerLab.com) is an independent testing organization that helps consumers learn more about product quality but requires an expensive subscription to obtain this information. Independent tests have found adulterants such as caffeine, indomethacin, prednisone, and pesticides in dietary supplements. Some acai berry supplements have been found to contain the prescription drug Viagra. Saper et al. (2008) analyzed 193 herbs and other dietary supplements manufactured in the United States and India and purchased on the Internet. Other test results indicate that 20 percent were contaminated with small amounts of heavy metals, including lead, mercury, and arsenic (Saper 2008). Since 1978, there have been reports of at least eighty cases of lead poisoning from Ayurvedic (Indian) medicine worldwide (Buettner 2009). As a buyer, you should beware. The FDA is taking steps to protect consumers from harm with dietary supplements used for weight loss, sexual enhancement, and body building. One step includes a new rapid-notification system to warn consumers about tainted supplements via the FDA's website (Cohen 2009).

The best way to find reliable information on the safety of dietary supplements is to have one central place to report and record unwanted side effects in the dietary-supplement industry (Shaw 2012). One such system exists for prescription and OTC medications in the United States and Europe, and it is starting to include supplements. Because herbs contain multiple constituents, side effects may be more difficult to quantify and qualify than those of prescription medications. Contributing factors to the amount and quality of active herbal-plant constituents include the plant's geographical origin, contents of the soil in which it was grown, parts of the plant that were harvested, when it was harvested, and where it was processed and stored.

No reference list is available to link all herbal plants and other dietary supplements by both the Latin scientific name and the common name. A project has been underway since 2012 to develop a "Medicinal Plants Names Index" at the Royal Botanic Gardens in Kew, England. This database will have cross-references of herbal names so herbal side effects can be reported internationally. The World Health Organization Collaborating Centre for Monitoring Drug Safety hopes to collate prescription medication, herbs, and other dietary-supplement adverse-reaction reports in one place.

Drug and Dietary-Supplement Interactions

Here are some examples of important, unsafe supplement and drug interactions to help you keep a healthy respect for this category of products (Matanovic 2012). Soy taken to lower cholesterol (or for its antioxidant value) can lessen the absorption of thyroid medications, such as Synthroid. St John's wort for depression can lessen the effectiveness of oral contraceptives. Garlic capsules and warfarin taken together can increase the risk of bruising and bleeding. Whole grapefruit, grapefruit juice, or grapeseed extract capsules can negatively interact with many prescription drugs, including those used for sleep, high cholesterol, heart-rhythm problems, pain, and hay fever (Fugh-Berman 2000). Remember, your pharmacist is an excellent resource for information concerning management of these interactions.

Dietary-Supplement Side Effects

In case you have not noticed, I am still trying just a wee bit to instill some fear into you about supplements. The Gallup Poll finds that year after year, pharmacists are among the most trusted healthcare professionals in the United States. We want to help.

Long-term ingestion of licorice (*Glycyrrhiza glabra*) can cause sodium and water to build up in the body. *Ephedra sinica* or ma huang may cause seizures, heart attack, and stroke. As an aside, *Ephedra sinica* was removed from the market for a while and now is more heavily regulated than in years past. Long-term use of ginkgo biloba, garlic (*Allium sativum*), vitamin E, ginger (*Zingiber officinale*), licorice (*Glycyrrhiza glabra*), and fish oil in higher doses may increase the risk of bruising and bleeding. Chaparral (*Larrea tridentate*), black cohosh (*Cimicifuga racemosa*), European mistletoe (*Viscum album*), kava kava (*Piper methysticum*), and valerian (*Valeriana officinalis*) may cause liver problems (Navarro 2009). Megadoses of vitamin A can increase the risk of hip fractures (Ramanathan 2009).

Under the right circumstances, herbs and other dietary supplements may enhance health. Products should be selected with the help of a pharmacist or a doctor who understands that supplements can be among many different evidence-based interventions for better health, as are prescription medications. Significant effects can be made by adopting a back-to-basics lifestyle consisting of good nutrition, sleep, and exercise as well as emotional, social, and spiritual health to stay well throughout life. In chapter 5 we will explore other complementary health and medicine interventions and start assembling a health tool kit.

CHAPTER 5

Complementary and Alternative Medicine: A Brave New World

> *The habitual use of any drug is harmful. The most eminent physicians are now agreed that very few drugs have any real curative value. The essential thing is right habits of life.*
> —John Harvey Kellogg

I met Marsha, a sixty-six-year-young woman, several years ago after giving a presentation to a group of community members. As a healthcare professional, Marsha understands the importance of balance. She expressed several of her health goals to me, including a desire to be whole-person balanced and to live a healthy lifestyle. Marsha wanted more wellness emphasis in her health regimen than her traditional-medicine doctor could offer. She was dealing with back pain, overuse of nonsteroidal anti-inflammatory drugs (NSAIDs), and depression. We agreed that healing could take place on multiple levels in her life journey and that it would require personal discipline, courage to move boldly into unknown territory, and a team of colleagues working together for her support. Evidence-based complementary and alternative medicine (CAM) seemed to be the likely next step in her list of potential interventions to achieve her stated health goals. Over time Marsha and I agreed that she could benefit from massage, laughter therapy, whole-food nutrition, a few dietary supplements, improved sleep habits, meaningful friendships outside of work, and daily meditation and deep breathing. Marsha loves to dance, but she was not dancing when we met because of her physical pain. I pray she is dancing today.

CAM is a combination of diverse practices and products that are not considered to be part of traditional medicine. Examples include acupuncture, massage, aromatherapy, and dietary supplements. Integrative medicine combines traditional and nontraditional practices. Alternative medicine is completely different from allopathic or traditional Western medicine. Holistic medicine is the art and science of healing that addresses the care of the whole person—body, mind, and spirit. The practice of holistic medicine integrates conventional and complementary therapies to promote optimal health and to prevent and treat disease by addressing its contributing factors. Where does my work fit into CAM? Although I call myself a holistic clinical pharmacist, my work integrates into and enhances recommendations from traditional medicine. There are many alternative-medicine practices that I do not believe are evidence based and that I believe can even cause harm.

A 2007 National Health Interview Survey (NHIS) of nearly twenty-four thousand adults at least eighteen years of age found that approximately 38 percent of adults are using some form of complementary or alternative medicine (Park 2008).

National thought leaders are talking about CAM. For three days in February 2009, nontraditional practitioners came together at the Institute of Medicine for the Summit on Integrative Health and the Health of the Public in Washington, DC. The summit was sponsored by the Bravewell Collaborative. More than six hundred scientists, top policy experts, healthcare industry leaders, and leading clinicians discussed practices and principles from integrative medicine that could affect healthcare reform in a positive way. They discussed how the patient is the center of care and that care should be focused on prevention and wellness, with body, mind, and spiritual needs taken into consideration. Participants considered that the progression of many chronic illnesses can be reversed and even completely healed through lifestyle modifications. Genetic inheritance is not our only health destiny. Our environment also influences health. Improving our primary-care and chronic-disease-care systems is paramount to moving the treatment paradigm toward prevention.

Since 2009, Surgeon General Regina Benjamin, MD, MBA, has chaired an advisory council to the National Prevention, Health Promotion, and Public Health Council that has developed a national healthcare strategy

(Benjamin 2013). Key initiatives detailed in this report include reducing prescription-drug abuse, improving nutrition, and encouraging healthy homelife. I wrote to Dr. Benjamin in 2011 and shared details about my professional philosophy and work. She embraced the concepts presented in this book and encouraged me to continue to educate others about them.

In addition to national legislative initiatives, changes in medical education are beginning to fuel practice patterns that incorporate wellness and prevention strategies into healthcare models such as the patient-centered medical home. The "home" represents a doctor-led, team-based care delivery model that provides thorough, ongoing care to its patients. The goal of this model is maximal health outcomes.

CAM has roots in Eastern tradition and practices. A prominent CAM practice, traditional Chinese medicine (TCM), focuses on whole-person balance and employs multimodal interventions. TCM focuses on symptoms that are signs of an imbalance caused by an unhealthy lifestyle or from an outside insult, such as infection or trauma. The imbalance is considered the root cause of the symptoms. TCM diagnostics include noninvasive pulse and tongue examination, different from American traditional-medicine invasive diagnostics and review of body systems and symptoms. Chinese diagnostics culminate in the practitioner assigning the patient to one or more categories of wind, water, wood, and fire—elements that represent imbalance in specific organ systems. Our forefathers did not have our technology, and external diagnostics made sense.

More than 130 countries use TCM, and 124 countries have Chinese medical institutes that offer TCM training, according to the Committee on Chinese Medicine and Pharmacy, Department of Health, Executive Yuan in Taiwan. TCM is growing at a rate of 10 percent a year.

By comparison, unique CAM programs are popping up in North America. For example, British Columbia has a program called the Complementary Medicine Education and Outcomes (CAMEO) program to help educate cancer patients and their healthcare professionals (Balneaves 2010). Table one shows some of the more popular CAM practices I have recommended to clients over the years.

Table 1—Examples of CAM Practices (Kessler 2001)

Practice and Description	More Information
Acupuncture: based on the principle that meridians of energy flow through the body. Blocked energy may need to be unblocked for overall health. Practitioners pierce the client's skin with thin needles manipulated by the practitioner's hands.	American Academy of Medical Acupuncture (medicalacupuncture.org)
Aromatherapy: use of essential oils to alter a person's mood or emotions. Some essential oils may have therapeutic properties.	National Association for Holistic Aromatherapy (naha.org)
Dietary supplements: includes vitamins, minerals, herbs, protein powders used in naturopathy, traditional Chinese medicine, Ayurveda, Kampo, and others.	Association of Natural Medicine Pharmacists (anmp.org)
Guided imagery: a technique that uses positive thoughts and images to stimulate the body's healing.	Academy for Guided Imagery (academyforguidedimagery.com) American Meditation Institute (americanmeditation.org)
Laughter therapy: the use of humor to promote overall emotional and physical health.	Association for Applied and Therapeutic Humor (aath.org)
Massage (LaStone, deep tissue, sports, neuromuscular, Swedish, craniosacral, shiatsu): involves manipulation of soft tissues and muscles.	American Massage Therapy Association (amtamassage.org)
Zumba: dance exercise emphasizing endurance and flexibility.	Zumba directory (zumba.com)
Music therapy: use of music to heal the emotions as guided by a music therapist.	American Music Therapy Association (musictherapy.org)
Spiritual practice: belief in a connection with nature or a higher power that motivates healthy principles for living such as forgiveness, service to others, and kindness.	Directory of retreat centers (findthedivine.com)

You may be a CAM skeptic. You may be wondering whether any nontraditional practices involve the placebo effect (Kaptchuk 2009). The placebo effect happens when patients engage in some type of intervention that they perceive will aid in healing, although the intervention has no proven therapeutic effect on the condition. This fascinating effect can happen with the use of prescription drugs, OTC drugs, dietary supplements, and nontraditional medicine practices (O'Connell 2009). Different types of placebos are used intentionally in research for the control group. Placebos, which are believed to work 30 percent of the time, contain no active ingredients (sugar pill) or active therapy (acupuncture needles placed improperly), but they still improve symptoms.

Some researchers believe that placebos cause psychological and physical responses. One such theory involves the subject-expectancy effect. When people already know what the result of taking a pill is supposed to be, they might report that result as the outcome even if they did not truly experience it. Other people have become classically conditioned to expect relief when they take medication. With both models, the client has an expectation. Chemical changes and susceptibility to the placebo effect might be genetically rooted.

By comparison, negative expectations are termed "the nocebo effect." Placebo and nocebo effects result from the psychosocial context of a medication or CAM intervention, or both, on the patient's body, mind, and spirit (Colloca 2012). Regardless of your belief about CAM therapies, safety is the first priority for all healthcare professionals. However, CAM therapies, including supplements, can cause unwanted effects. Adverse-event reporting related to a broad spectrum of CAM interventions is complicated but necessary to protect consumers around the world. If you try any CAM therapies and experience an unwanted effect, please report it to your CAM practitioner as well as to your doctor for directions on how to manage it.

Do you want to try a CAM intervention but are hesitant to talk with your doctor about it? Start by searching for a doctor who is open to working with a team of CAM practitioners. Then choose among the more than two hundred CAM practices available in the United States. Remember, not all of them are evidence based. Be sensitive to the fact that your doctor might be wary about referring you to CAM because any negative outcomes ultimately would reflect back onto the physician or could cause you harm.

Here are some things to remember when selecting a CAM practitioner:

- Check with your doctor or pharmacist for a referral to an evidence-based CAM practitioner. Make sure the practice is safe and effective for your specific condition.
- Gather information on CAM practitioners in your area before you visit one. Ask office staff or the practitioner about training, years of experience, and credentials—such as academic degrees, certification, competencies, registration, licensure, and apprenticeship.
- Contact a national or state professional organization for the type of practitioner you are seeking. Ask whether that particular practitioner specializes in any health conditions.
- Find out whether the therapy you seek is covered by your health insurance. Most CAM interventions are not covered by insurance.
- List questions you wish to ask your CAM practitioner at your first visit. Examples include the benefits and risks you could expect from the therapy, how long you would need to undergo treatment, whether the practitioner has scientific literature supporting the therapy, how many patients the practitioner has treated with the same types of symptoms as yours, and what the practitioner's success rate is for healing.
- Most important, disclose all CAM visits to your doctor so your overall health and wellness care may be coordinated for optimal outcomes.

If you are not satisfied or comfortable with your CAM practitioner, seek out a different one or discontinue CAM treatment if professionally advised. No harm will come to you in the process.

In chapter 6 we will talk in more detail about a CAM model I have designed called the Eight-Balance-Point Model for Healing. This model has evolved over many years and came from hours of listening to people share their personal health journeys and unmet needs. What a privilege it is, and what a blessing to be in that healing space with others.

CHAPTER 6

Personalized Health and Wellness: The Eight-Balance-Point Model for Healing

> *Nobody can go back and start a new beginning, but anyone can start today and make a new ending.*
> —Maria Robinson

Mark is a seventy-two-year-young man who was referred to me by his oncologist. I first met him when he was a few years out from a radical prostatectomy and radiation for cancer. I continued to work with him as a member of his handpicked CAM team of professionals, as well as another group of traditional doctors and specialists around the country. Mark's ultimate goal was to halt cancer growth and improve his quality of life. Mark tracked his prostate-specific antigen (PSA)—a marker used to follow cancer progression or remission—and showed me that it was rising. Mark was a former fitness buff and was dealing with acid-reflux disease and business-related stress. He would send me published literature on more controversial therapies to treat resistant prostate cancer, including various foods, OTC medications, and dietary supplements. I was asked to evaluate each test tube or animal study and give him my professional opinion about whether or not he should try the interventions, with permission from his doctors. We talked about his supplement intake for general and immune health and how that strategy was to be combined with his anticancer strategy to avoid duplication or unwanted interactions. To say that Mark's outlook on life and take-charge personality positively affected his journey would be an understatement. The CAM interventions he tried delayed his disease progression for some time, but it did not achieve the outcome he desired. Yet through the time that I knew Mark, I can honestly say he claimed his body, mind, and spiritual blessings about which I have spoken in a previous chapter—a house, food on the table, family, friends, freedom to worship, and a good job.

Many times during our professional conversations, he gave me a rare glimpse into what it was like to suffer from a chronic illness and how unresolved emotional and spiritual issues affect coping mechanisms. We talked more about faith than most people are comfortable doing during a consultation. It was in those precious moments that I was privileged to witness the heartfelt emotions that every person will experience sooner or later on this earth. These opportunities prepared me for what I had to endure when my mother passed away from an extended illness. Mark's story was inspirational. He demonstrated to me that he was spiritually ready to change.

Readiness to Change

Although searching for more sustainable ways to achieve optimal health may seem intuitive, it's hard for most of us in the autumn of life to change longtime habits and take our complicated lifestyles back to the basics. Yet a well-thought-out healing plan is essential to achieving abundant joy in our journey and is part of being able to live life to its fullest with purpose and peace. We plan for other important times in life, such as vacations, college, and retirement. It makes perfect sense to add a plan for health and wellness to that important list of to-dos (Norcross 2011).

Here is an example of how to go about it. First, if you do not want to or cannot go on a CAM hunt yourself, as we discussed in the previous chapter, find a healthcare advocate such as an integrative doctor, pharmacist, or nurse who can help select and coordinate your CAM team and will be in charge of overseeing and triaging your overall care. This advocate may be your primary-care doctor. The team's composition might depend on what aspects of body, mind, and spiritual health you wish to focus.

Next, cultivate your own personal characteristics of accountability and discipline, and make a commitment to change. Address any ambivalence to change, including your fears, any reluctance to take risks, or any disbelief in your ability to achieve your health goals. Set aside time to prioritize health changes. Find a mentor, coach, or encourager to hold you accountable for the decisions you make.

All of life involves change, yet many people find change uncomfortable. You may not be ready at this time of your life just because someone else wants you to improve your health habits. Change comes in stages: being aware of the need to change, thinking about change, preparing to change, and making the change. Celebrate small gains, but be prepared to slip from time to time until you achieve your ultimate goal. Where are you now? Where would you like to be in six months? One year? Five years? These are important questions you must answer first.

The April 16, 2012, edition of *The Wall Street Journal* had an article about transforming healthcare by focusing on quality of life. Authors published results from the Centers for Disease Control and Prevention 2008 Survey on adults, conducted by Porter Novelli, regarding their overall health. Of those surveyed 15 percent said they felt calm and peaceful all the time within the previous thirty days. Only 19 percent strongly agreed that they were satisfied with their lives, and 11 percent felt cheerful all the time in the previous thirty days. You might wonder about the kinds of lives these folks are leading. Maybe some need the Eight-Balance-Point Model for Healing to light their paths. Others might benefit from a bucket, rag, soap, and water to start their life-cleansing process.

When you are ready to establish your health goals, the Eight-Balance-Point Model for Healing is a framework that can be used as a template to begin implementing change. The eight balance points include interventions for physical health, healthy nutrition and supplements, exercise, restorative sleep, emotional health, relationship health, environmental health, and spiritual health. Think of them as steps on your health ladder. The top rung of your ladder is spiritual health. Let's examine each one of these balance points in detail.

Physical Health

This aspect of whole-person health is directed by our primary-care doctors, who prescribe preventive, diagnostic laboratory, and other tests. Routine tests for normal-risk adults, as published by the US Department of Health and Human Services, check blood pressure, weight and nutritional intake, PAP smears for women, blood-cholesterol levels, fasting blood-sugar levels, mammograms for women only, colonoscopies after age fifty, vision, hearing, thyroid, CBC, metabolic panel, PSA (men only), and skin-cancer screening. Also important are immunization shots for tetanus, pertussis, diphtheria, measles, mumps, rubella, pneumococcal disease, influenza, and hepatitis B. Your primary-care doctor also will provide counseling with regard to bone health, including nutrition; weight-bearing exercise; calcium, vitamin D, and vitamin K2 intake; tobacco use; and alcohol use. A few doctors will talk with you about their concerns regarding polypharmacy. Choose a primary-care doctor to be the gatekeeper for your overall wellness plan, and keep regular office appointments. Ask about ways to take prescription medications less frequently when appropriate. Consider incorporating CAM therapies when appropriate. More than two hundred types of CAM therapies are practiced in the United States, most of which are not covered by third-party insurance or Medicare.

Nutrition and Dietary Supplements

Whole foods were placed on the earth as fuel for our nourishment. Consumerism has overpackaged and genetically modified our food. We should resist fast or processed food and try to eat foods in their natural states as much as possible. Dietary supplements have roles alongside whole nutrition, but are not intended to replace healthy food choices. Start every day with breakfast. Eat small snacks frequently during the day instead of two or three large meals. Take a cooking class or a class on general nutrition. Many high-end grocery stores provide this service. Grow an organic vegetable garden. Is there anything better than a fresh, homegrown tomato? Add plants, nuts, beans, fish, low-fat dairy products, colorful fruits and vegetables, and healthy monounsaturated and polyunsaturated oils to your diet. Read about the Mediterranean diet, the world's gold standard to healthy nutrition, which has been studied head-to-head with the American Heart Association's recommended low-fat diet and found to be superior in preventing heart disease (Kris-Etherton 2001).

Adding protein and antioxidant-rich food to your diet helps build a strong immune system. Examples of healthy protein are fish, lean chicken breasts, turkey, beans, nuts, and low-fat dairy products.

Antioxidant-rich foods include blueberries, cherries, broccoli, cauliflower, tomatoes, onions, acai berries, pomegranate, kiwis, artichokes, and decaffeinated green tea. Examples of antioxidant chemical classes are polyphenols (flavonoids) and carotenoids. Flavonoids include catechin, apigenin, quercetin, anthocyanidins, astaxanthin, and zeaxanthin. Use each of these in a sentence at your next dinner party and impress the beta carotene out of your guests. Eating whole foods provides so much more health value with the thousands of antioxidant constituents in plants provided in nature than taking one dietary supplement—such as a vitamin—out of a bottle.

Anti-inflammatory foods and spices may help keep your joints and blood vessels lubricated. Anti-inflammatory foods include fish oil; oily fish such as salmon, herring, and sardines; walnuts; cold-pressed extra-virgin olive oil; canola oil; curry; avocado; and herbs and spices, such as ginger, rosemary, oregano, turmeric, and parsley.

Foods such as oatmeal, cinnamon, soy, and artichokes help keep blood-cholesterol levels low. Foods that are low on the glycemic index help balance blood sugar. Gluten-free foods help manage wheat or rye allergies. Foods in the DASH diet help reduce blood-sodium content to manage high blood pressure. Whenever you can afford them and they are available, purchase locally grown organic whole foods so you know what's on your family's table. Season your food with more herbs and spices instead of salt.

Do not exceed the daily recommended doses for fat-soluble vitamins— A, D, E, and K—because they can accumulate in the body. High doses of vitamin A over the long term increase the risk of hip fractures (Caire-Juvera 2009). It is better to eat carrots for their vitamin-A content contributing to eye health. Excessive doses of vitamin E have been associated with an increased risk of stroke (visit http://www.mayoclinic.org/drugs-supplements/vitamin-e/safety/HRB-20060476). Vitamin D is the sunshine vitamin and contributes to bone health, but too much vitamin D out of the bottle may cause nonspecific symptoms such as weakness, fatigue, dry mouth, sleepiness, headache, and loss of appetite.

A safe rule of thumb is to not exceed 200 percent of the recommended daily allowance for all vitamins and minerals—especially those that are fat soluble—unless otherwise directed by your doctor. Remember, supplements cannot replace good eating habits.

If you live in a larger city, try to find a food co-op or a consumer-supported agriculture farm (CSA) near you, develop a good working relationship with a farmer, and share in the crops. Check out farmers' markets in your area.

Seek out organic milk from cows that have not been fed antibiotics or hormones. Better yet, choose milk and chicken from organic farms. Almond milk is a good source of calcium if you do not like the taste of cow's milk, although it has less protein per serving than cow's milk.

Exercise

Our bodies are built to move, not to remain seated for most of the day at a desk. In addition to movement, regular exercise is a key component to health. Talk with your doctor to be sure you are able to handle exercise. Then choose an exercise accountability partner who wants to stay healthy and exercise just like you do and remind you when you are not acting on your promise to work out. A personal trainer is best if you have the time and can afford one. Walking or biking in nature is free and an excellent way to start moving.

Research recommends thirty minutes of strenuous exercise to one hour of moderate exercise most days of the week. This can be done in several time portions or all at once. The important thing is that you try. Look for ways to include exercise focused on endurance, muscle strength, flexibility, balance, and bone strength. Pilates is a workout that focuses on your core strength. If you are adventuresome, Zumba, hiking, canoeing, in-line skating, roller skating, skiing, and swimming are options. You may include stretching for limber muscles, weight lifting for strength training and bone density, or running for endurance. Start slowly, ten to fifteen minutes a day, and build up gradually as time and endurance permit. Develop a routine that fits your lifestyle.

Movement keeps the veins open and prevents clots in your legs. Motion keeps arteries pumping with oxygen to your tissues and organs.

Step aerobics are good for the heart. Research indicates that exercise helps keep your heart muscle strong.

Restorative Sleep

It's so important to get enough sleep on a regular basis. Most people need seven to eight hours every night. The older we get, the harder it may be to sleep. For women this becomes more problematic after menopause. Here are a few medication-free, holistic tips to help fall asleep and remain asleep through the night:

- Before retiring, drink a glass of warm milk with a half teaspoon of nutmeg on top, or a cup of decaffeinated green tea. Milk, chamomile tea (*Matricaria recutita*), lavender tea (*Lavendula angustifolia*), purple bee balm tea (*Monarda didyma*), and decaffeinated green tea contain relaxing constituents.
- Empty your bladder before retiring so there is less need to get up in the middle of the night to go to the bathroom.
- Write down a list of unfinished business and some of your major worries from the day on a piece of paper, and put the paper somewhere away from the bedroom. Part with these thoughts until tomorrow, for tomorrow is another day.
- Keep the temperature in the bedroom cool. A cooler room increases the body's natural melatonin level, which helps induce sleep.
- Place a small drop of lavender (*lavandula angustifolia*) essential oil on your pillow as a relaxing fragrance (aromatherapy).
- Upon retiring, breathe deeply in and out evenly for five minutes while reciting a list of blessings out loud or in your mind.
- Do some light stretching before bedtime to relax your muscles.
- Play soft instrumental music or music with nature sounds before bedtime.
- If you enjoy reading, pick up a book before bedtime.
- Dreaming is indicative of the deepest rapid-eye-movement (REM) sleep and indicates that we have had a good night's sleep. Strive for restorative sleep with dreams.

Emotional Health

Where our thoughts go, so do our emotions (Goleman 1998). Repeating affirming thoughts can help us cope with depression, anxiety, and fears. This easy technique can change negative thoughts into positive ones. For parents it is also important to affirm our children for who they are, not for what they do. Examples of affirming statements can express that you are lovable, healthy, whole, blessed, forgiven, fortunate, or thankful.

Examining our thoughts helps us identify trends and patterns and avoid situations that trigger negative thinking. Meditation and guided imagery are two CAM practices that emphasize the mind-body connection and help us stay in the present to clear our minds. We can have emotional healing even if physical symptoms of chronic illness persist. Practice a few minutes of slow, deep breathing. Sit up straight in your chair with good posture. Inhale through your nose to the count of five, hold the breath for just a moment, and exhale through your mouth to the count of five. Repeat two to three times. Notice how good you feel after this exercise and how the life-giving oxygen flowing through your nostrils refreshes you.

Goleman speaks about competencies in our emotional intelligence (1998). Emotional accountability includes self-awareness and self-control. Self-awareness comes from recognizing the consequences of our emotions and reviewing our emotional strengths and weaknesses.

Next is the Myers-Briggs Type Indicator personality profile (Briggs Myers 1995). Taking this test helps you become aware of how you process information, react in calm and in stressful moments, and relate to others. Four pairs of preferences were taken from Carl Jung's psychological theories from the early 1920s and are categorized as follows: extroversion or introversion, sensing or intuition, thinking or feeling, and judgment or perception. Our personalities can change over time.

The DISC assessment is another behavioral model based on the work of psychologist William Moulton Martson, PhD, in the late nineteenth and early twentieth centuries. DISC describes four personality profiles. D stands for dominance, I is for influence, S is for steadiness, and C is for compliance. D types shape the environment by overcoming opposition and challenge. I types shape the environment by persuading and influencing others. S types achieve stability and accomplish tasks by cooperating with others, and C types work within circumstances to ensure quality and accuracy.

According to Martson, understanding each of these types, including your own, can contribute to the health of personal relationships as well as work teams.

Finally, there is the Enneagram, with nine types of personalities or points of view on how we react to people and life situations (Palmer 1995). According to Palmer, "the perfectionist" searches for perfection, has high moral character, and wants to do right and be right. "The giver" needs others' approval and wants to be needed. "The performer" is focused on goals, tasks, and productiveness. "The romantic" seems to always want what is unavailable, is melancholy, and may be called a "drama queen" or "drama king." "The observer" is preoccupied with privacy, knowledge, independence, and emotional control. "The trooper" is a procrastinator who sometimes does not complete goals, has authority problems, and identifies with the underdogs in life. "The epicure" craves stimulating activities, hedges commitment, and uses charm as a first line of defense. "The boss" wants to control personal space and possessions, is concerned about justice and power, and denies personal weakness. "The mediator" avoids conflict, has ambivalence about personal decisions, does not like change, and can't say no.

In summary, we all have traits of several personality types, usually with one or two dominating. Regardless of which technique you use to better understand your emotions, I hope you will take a moment to reflect on your emotional maturity in challenging situations. Think about how you react under stress. Do you think before you speak? An entire chapter in this book is devoted to stress management.

Laughing frequently is also important to your emotional health. Can we ever laugh too much? Laughter can ease our worries and stress and is good for the soul. It provides a workout for muscles and unleashes stress-busting endorphins or painkillers into the bloodstream. Laughter therapists help people laugh more easily (Brown 2011). Laughter doesn't come easily to everyone, but the body cannot distinguish between real and fake laughter. Have you heard about laughter yoga? What will they think of next?

Relationship Health

We live in a high-tech, low-touch, low face-to-face-interaction society. Time spent in loving relationships with family, platonic friends, romantic love interests, and animals helps us feel complete. Animals teach us unconditional love, something we all want but is sometimes hard to find. Seek out friendships with people who are nonjudgmental, are good listeners, and can accept you the way you are. Try to accept others as they are. A universal nurturing sisterhood among women develops after our children are raised and move out of the house, after our parents pass on, and after other life transitions. When retirement comes, men may bond with male friends through breakfast gatherings, Bible studies, or golf dates. Seek out such a women's or men's group near you. Talk with individuals who are lonely, volunteer to help with meal preparation and delivery for shut-in people, and get involved in other service-oriented activities that focus on community health. In turn, your health will be improved. Think about writing letters to friends you have not seen for some time. Become a pen pal to a service member in active duty.

Environmental Health

Are you mindful of the unhealthy things to which you are exposed every day? These can include the dry-cleaning chemicals on our clothes, the estrogen-containing pesticides on our lawns, chemicals in deodorants and hair sprays, microwaves from the oven, radiation from cell phones, chlorinated water, and aluminum in antiperspirants. Making a conscious choice to avoid some of these toxins can be daunting, but there are always options. It can be done and is worth the extra money for your long-term health. For starters, consider organic herbicides for your lawn, organic milk from cows not fed growth-enhancing hormones or unnecessary antibiotics, and natural deodorants that do not contain aluminum.

Spiritual Health

Our physical body will change throughout life. That realization has emotional and spiritual implications (Ludwig 2008). Where do we learn about spiritual health? Outside of churches, synagogues, and mosques, nature and the universe send us spiritual messages all day long. I'm convinced that a fulfilling and joyous life can be maintained through life's trials by focusing on our spiritual selves and spending more time in nature. Unstructured outdoor play fosters creative energy all the way through life, not just when we are children. Consider how easy it is to be childlike in your relationships with grandchildren. That same energy edifies boomers. Employ all of your senses—sight, taste, hearing, touch, and smell—during playtime. The senses can evoke positive emotions and help us heal. Smile. Look for miracles. Miracles happen every day to those who are open to them.

Tools for spiritual health include regular prayer, forgiveness, worship, servant leadership, and being intentional about our life purpose.

Prayer

Spiritual messages come from that still voice inside us. As a Christian I believe the voice is the Holy Spirit. Belief in the power of prayer can be reassuring and spiritually satisfying. Prayer can take place directly between the believer and a higher power in private or through others interceding on one's behalf (Kuchan 2008). I frequently ask permission to pray with or for a client at the close of our consulting sessions because it creates a safe place filled with trust and care (Rosenbaum 2007).

Forgiveness

Imagine swallowing your pride, picking up the phone, and calling a former friend with whom you have not spoken for many years because of a falling-out. Imagine starting the conversation by saying, "I am sorry," and asking for forgiveness for whatever it was that caused the falling-out. The person on the other end of the phone will feel something. That is certain. Both parties will immediately feel that a weight has been lifted and sense happiness, even if just for that brief moment. You will feel this even if the recipient is not happy about the experience. Where our thoughts go, so do our emotions. A number of years ago, I reached out to my best girlfriend from high school with whom I had not spoken in more than thirty years. I asked her to forgive me for not including her in my wedding and not staying in touch. She was gracious and loving, and we have remained in contact ever since. What a blessing for us both. We remain close friends because of that one simple step in faith.

Worship

I highly recommend the book *The Blue Zones* by Dan Buettner. Dan is an American explorer and educator who has visited five areas of the world where people live to be at least one hundred years old. According to Dan, two of the common bonds are that these people have a strong sense of family and regularly attend worship in a venue of their choice.

Servant Leadership

We cannot become trusted leaders until we first serve others in business or in our family life. Positive spiritual thoughts also may have a role in clinical practice (Larimore 2002; O'Hara 2002). Robert Greenleaf writes about learning to relate to one another in "creatively supportive" instead of dictatorial ways (Greenleaf 2002). Relating engenders good listening skills and a willingness to sacrifice time for the good of others while maintaining boundaries to avoid compassion fatigue.

Life Purpose

This is usually not the main topic of discussion at the family dinner table, but it may be interesting to talk with a close friend about defining spirituality and how it connects to a life legacy. Another way to leave a legacy to future generations begins with exploring your spiritual self with a trusted spiritual mentor—a pastor, a rabbi, or other member of clergy. Spiritual research and spiritual retreats are other options for growth and will be covered in more detail in chapter 9 (Jonas 2001).

> *When everything seems to be going against you, remember that the airplane takes off against the wind, not with it.*
> —Henry Ford

Healthy Changes Can Begin Today

Now that we have laid the foundation for the Eight-Balance-Point Model for Healing, let's discuss some of the CAM interventions in more detail. The remaining chapters will focus on CAM practices that are evidence based and can be used to improve your health. Remember that you can be an equal partner on your integrative health and medicine team that includes recommendations for, and access to, these types of interventions.

CHAPTER 7
Combating Superstress with Guided Imagery

> *When you stop giving, when you stop offering*
> *something to someone, it's time to turn out the light.*
> —GEORGE BURNS

Carol came to see me at a particularly vulnerable time in her life. She was well into the process of completing her master's degree, and she was dealing with chronic health issues. Her significant other wanted to spend more time with her. Their different life needs caused a major decline in her overall health and energy level. Carol was burned out. She took out her frustrations in food and gained weight. She had no time to enjoy nature, and she found walking any distance difficult because of chronic joint pain. We explored guided imagery as one viable tool to reduce stress. I have thought about Carol many times. Her story is common. It is a wake-up call to slow down.

In today's fast-paced business world and in many overscheduled families, superstress is created over time. Stress may not be recognized until a physical ailment manifests itself or sleep is compromised. Although it is a subjective experience, stress is basically an emotional and physical response to life's challenges and changes. Perhaps the psychological aspects of stress outweigh the physical in the short term, but in the long term they can rob us of overall health.

Causes of Stress—The Holmes and Rahe Stress Scale

In 1967 psychiatrists Thomas Holmes and Richard Rahe determined that stress contributes to illness. Around that time, Rahe validated the scale as a predictor of illness by administering it to a group of US sailors who were asked to rate the scores of their "life events" over the prior six months. From this study, Rahe found that significant life changes contributing to stress include death of a spouse, divorce, personal illness, losing a job, retirement, sex difficulties, financial problems, and post-traumatic stress disorder. These events can be the root causes of many symptoms affecting quality of life. Sooner or later, at least one of these events will be part of most people's lives.

Signs and Symptoms of Superstress

Muscle-tension headaches	Difficulty sleeping
Teeth grinding	Forgetfulness
Muscle aches (neck, back)	Irritability, hostility, anger
Heartburn, stomach pain	Social withdrawal
Constipation, diarrhea	Increased smoking, alcohol use
Panic attack	Immune suppression
Chest pain, high blood pressure	Rapid heart rate
Anxiety, depression	Difficulty in making decisions
Change in appetite	Reduced work productivity

Mind-Body Connection and Stress

Have you heard of the mind-body connection? Here is how it works. The brain releases a hormone to the pituitary. Then the pituitary releases another hormone, adrenocorticotropic hormone (ACTH), into the blood. ACTH activates the adrenal gland to release cortisol into the blood, and the brain activates the adrenal gland to release epinephrine and norepinephrine—fight-or-flight chemicals—causing an increase in natural opioids for pain relief during extremely stressful situations. However, long-term elevation of cortisol promotes nerve death in the brain, suppresses the immune system, and can impair insulin regulation. Not good. Although humans can experience lots of stress in life, zebras apparently do not. I recommend *Why Zebras Don't Get Ulcers*, by Robert Sapolsky, for a good laugh. Maybe we should be more like these creatures and adopt their outlook on life. On a more serious note, let's take a look at some of the most common stress-related symptoms and what we can do about them from a noninvasive perspective.

Muscle Tension, Headache, and Neck and Back Pain

Tension headaches can be caused by tight muscles in the back of the neck and scalp, resulting from poor posture, anxiety, or insufficient sleep. Try getting a massage, which has been shown to decrease cortisol levels and relax tired muscles. At work take frequent breaks from sitting at a computer or desk. Ask your employer for an ergonomic assessment and office setup to ensure good body mechanics while sitting for long periods.

When the sympathetic fight-or-flight system in the body is activated during stress, more blood is delivered to muscles to help the body flee the situation if danger prevails. Walking and talking out our daily problems helps calm us and reduce muscle tension.

Chest Pain

Chest pain can be caused by reduced blood flow to the heart arteries, gastrointestinal pain, or anxiety. Regardless of the perceived cause, report any chest pain to your doctor right away. A medical doctor should make the diagnosis and treat the pain. Deep breathing for five minutes in the middle of the stressful moment is one method to reduce chest pain caused by anxiety, chronic stress, and fear.

Anger and Hostility

Try to recognize the physical manifestations of anger when it happens and focus on calming down. Listen to your body, and be aware of your anger. Anger and rage are toxic emotions. Taking a time-out from the situation may be warranted to cool off and cope. Talk therapy for anger management, deep breathing for a few minutes, or watching a funny movie or reading a funny book as time permits may help.

Change in Appetite

Superstress, sleep deprivation, and an increased appetite are all linked and influenced by the duration of the stress and the coping mechanism of each person. Try to get restorative sleep for seven to eight hours each night. If appetite increases from lack of sleep, switch from three large meals each day to grazing with frequent, healthy snacks such as fruits and vegetables.

Gastrointestinal and Immune Symptoms

Both the small and large intestines can be affected by stress. Overactive small intestines react with constipation. Overactive large intestines react with chronic diarrhea or inflammatory bowel disease. Guided imagery, deep breathing, and other relaxation techniques are good interventions to help manage these symptoms. An overworked immune system is depressed by stress, and this increases the risk of illness. Probiotic foods, protein, and antioxidant foods all contribute to immunity health. Increasing fibrous foods and water intake will counteract constipation.

Guided Imagery

Of the various CAM interventions discussed in this chapter, guided imagery is my favorite and best illustrates the mind-body connection. Thanks to the research of Irving Oyle, the Simontons, and Roberto Assagioli, guided imagery has been practiced since the 1970s. Techniques include simple visualization and direct suggestion with mental imagery as well as storytelling. A certified guided-imagery practitioner instructs the student to think of a pleasant mental image and to pay attention to any emotions and senses relative to that image. After a few sessions, the student learns to imagine pleasant scenes independently through repeated visualization. The student draws on inner resources—such as the senses—to creatively work through stress and other health challenges.

In Sarah Ban Breathnach's book *Simple Abundance: A Daybook of Comfort and Joy, Sensory Awakening,* we read that Oscar Wilde said, "Nothing can cure the soul but the senses, just as nothing can cure the senses but the soul."

Guided imagery is an evidence-based CAM practice. Research with the positron emission tomography (PET) scanner demonstrates that parts of the brain are similarly activated when we simply *imagine* a scene as when we actually *experience* that scene. Guided imagery allows the student to relax and focus on mental images associated with health issues they want to confront and move past. In medical terms, imagining a picture sends a message to the limbic system—where our emotions originate—and then to the autonomic nervous system and to the immune system. People coping with stress-related problems—such as high blood pressure and a rapid heart rate—can be asked to imagine a place where there is no stress. The guided-imagery practitioner encourages the student to find creative solutions to relax (Schaffer 2013; Boehm 2013; Menzies 2014).

A word of caution is in order for anyone with a diagnosis of psychosis or a borderline personality disorder. Guided imagery is not intended to replace care with a licensed psychologist or psychiatrist.

The Academy for Guided Imagery (Acadgi.com) provides certification training for this CAM practice. Visit HolisticOnline.com, GuidedImageryInc.com, or Ami-BonnyMethod.org for more information.

CHAPTER 8
Aromatherapy: Lavender's Blue (Dilly, Dilly)

> *Hot lavender, mints, savory, marjoram;*
> *The marigold, that goes to bed wi' th' sun,*
> *And with him rises weeping; these are flow'rs*
> *Of middle summer, and I think they are given*
> *To men of middle age.*
> —Shakespeare from *The Winter's Tale*

Aromatherapy is the use of plant essences to affect or alter a person's mood in order to facilitate physical, mental, and emotional well-being and to manage stress (Papadopoulos 1999, Soo Lee 2012, Cooke 2000). From ancient Egyptian times to the modern age, essential oils have been used for health and well-being. Oils were popularized in biblical times for embalming and anointing and were reintroduced for therapeutic and recreational use in 1928 by the French chemist Rene-Maurice Gattefosse.

Volatile essential oils, distilled from plant extracts, have small molecular structures, which allows them to penetrate the skin and be absorbed into the bloodstream and lymph system. When inhaled, essential oils send a signal to the limbic system via neurochemicals in the brain through a direct connection to olfactory bulb nerves in the nose (Bent 2000).

There is no standard definition for the term "therapeutic aromatherapy." Topical use of essential oils for stress reduction and improved sleep has been described in the literature (Setzer 2009). Seek a qualified healthcare professional prior to using essential oils for topical indications, especially if you are pregnant, are elderly, or have asthma, epilepsy, or heart disease. Testing on the sole of the foot is recommended prior to first use to determine sensitivity and allergic potential. If irritation develops, discontinue use.

The extraction process, including distillation and expression, must be precise to ensure high-quality products. Do your homework when selecting a particular brand of essential oils. The table below outlines the dilution methods. Do not keep *homemade* combination ingredients or products longer than one month before discarding them and preparing a fresh batch of the final product.

Use and Amount of Essential Oil	Dilution Instructions
Massage: three or four drops	One teaspoonful of olive, jojoba, or sesame oil (your choice for homemade massage oil)
Foot bath; two drops	Four liters (four quarts) of warm water
Pillow sachet, handkerchief, candle fragrance: one or two drops	Undiluted
Infuser: five or six drops	Undiluted
Liquid bubble bath: one drop	Eight-ounce bottle of product
Vacuum cleaner bag: three or four drops	Undiluted

Topical essential oils placed on the skin can cause contact dermatitis and skin irritation because of aldehyde or phenol content, such as from thyme (*Thymus vulgaris*), oregano (*Origanum vulgare*), or cinnamon (*Cinnamomum cassia*). To avoid irritation, dilute the oils before applying them sparingly to the skin. Some oils are light-sensitive and should be used only indoors or at night. These include the citrus oils lime (*Citrus aurantifolia*), lemon (*Citrus limon*), and sweet orange (*Citrus sinensis*). Always store essential oils in their original containers, away from direct sunlight, and keep them out of the reach of children. Keep essential oils away from the eyes. Discard any undiluted essential oils in their original containers every few weeks (up to three months) and repurchase fresh products for topical use, properly diluted in vegetable oil.

Lavender

Essential oils can evoke our emotions to help us imagine a place of peace. Lavender is a versatile essential oil and can be used to enhance sleep, to relax, and to relieve stress. There are many species of lavender, a perennial plant from the mint family (Fismer 2012). Research them. Lavender works well in combination with other essential oils.

Synergistic Essential Oil Blends for Inhalation	
Meditation	Frankincense (*Boswellia serrata*), lavender (*Lavandula angustifolia*), sandalwood (*Santalum album*)
Relaxation (Setzer 2009)	Rosewood (*Aniba rosaeodora*), jasmine (*Jasminum officinale*), rose (*Rosa damascena*), jonquil (*Narcissus jonquilla*)
Sleep (Sarris 2001)	Mandarin (*Citrus reticulata*), lavender (*Lavandula angustifolia*), lemon (*Citrus limon*), dill (*Anethum graveolens*)
Stress relief (Sayorwan 2012)	Sandalwood (*Santalum album*), lavender (*Lavandula angustifolia*), grapefruit (*Citrus paradisi*)
Uplifting mood	Mandarin (*Citrus reticulata*), lime (*Citrus aurantifolia*), rosewood (*Aniba rosaeodora*), eucalyptus (*Eucalyptus globulus*), orange (*Citrus sinensis*)
Postoperative nausea (Hunt 2013)	Ginger (*Zingiber officinale*), spearmint (*Mentha spicata*), peppermint (*Mentha piperita*), cardamom (*Elettaria cardamomum*)

CHAPTER 9
Spiritual Renewal: Exploring Life's Mysteries

Quiet the mind, and the soul will speak.
—MA JAYA SATI BHAGAVATI, FROM *THE 11 KARMIC SPACES: CHOOSING FREEDOM FROM THE PATTERNS THAT BIND YOU*

We will end on the aspect of spirituality—that ongoing relationship with God or a higher power, regardless of whether one is physically and emotionally healthy or unhealthy. No universal definition for spirituality exists (Ledger 2005), yet spiritual awareness is essential to our very being (Tuck 2006; Oman 2006).

Regarding the acute healing process in athletes, studies have shown that adding elements of spirituality improves injury management and overall recovery (McKnight 2001). Depression management and improved coping with serious medical illness have been associated with spirituality or religious practices (Williams 2014). Struve reports that patients experienced healing through prayer at some time in their lives and valued doctors' inclusions of spiritual questions as a more comprehensive source of encouragement (Struve 2002).

At the beginning of this book, you learned that my dad's healing defied logic and science and clearly included a spiritual dimension. Our family agreed that God was on Dad's team guiding his outcome. "Spiritual dimension is the most direct experience of the universal life force" (Thornton 2005). What does spirituality look like, and what tools are needed to achieve spiritual growth and healing in addition to what we have covered in chapter 6? One tool involves creating a spiritual journal and taking a spiritual-gifts inventory to explore our areas of strength and then testing them with others. Spiritual gifts are identified by Paul in the Bible in Romans 12:4–8, Ephesians 4:7–12, and 1 Corinthians 12:7–11 and 27–30. Examples are prophecy, serving, teaching, exhortation, leadership, discernment, and evangelism. Visit http://mintools.com/spiritual-gifts-test.htm for more information about the test. Natural talents can be used for any purpose, but God-given spiritual gifts are to help us connect with our higher power. Spiritual inventory also includes exploring various heart aspects of your journey.

Shepherd's Heart

Our mind can be likened to a shepherd's heart. Turn that shepherding instinct inward, and continue to dream, to envision, and to reinvent yourself throughout life. People's reach for growth should exceed their grasp of present state throughout life.

Steward's Heart

A steward's heart can represent our body. Our bodies are temples, and we are caretakers of these temples. Nutrition, sleep, and regular exercise build strong bodies with evolved senses, resonating with the power of touch. A March 10, 2008, article in *The Wall Street Journal* gave us this headline: "A Touch of Grace: Massage Therapy Aids Retired Nuns. Bronx Nursing Home Finds Drug Alternative." Here are the first few lines: "Turns out one Harold Packman (85 years young) has developed an important expertise: giving massages to women who may have spent a lifetime shying away from this kind of physical contact. This is heaven to the nuns." Providence Nursing Home hired Harold, a licensed massage therapist, as part of an unusual experiment to cut their use of restraints and antipsychotic medications to sedate agitated patients. The nursing home developed regimens involving aromatherapy, soothing bubble baths, and Harold's massages. The result? Although some 30 percent of nursing-home patients nationwide are put on antipsychotics, Providence has reduced that number from 23 percent of its residents to 2 percent with these programs. From this story we can learn about the importance of stewardship as well as massage.

Servant's Tender Heart

Emotions are likened to a servant's tender heart. Where our authentic thoughts go, so do our emotions. The twelve-step program for Alcoholics Anonymous (12step.org) encourages participants to make a list of people they have harmed, to ask for forgiveness from them, to hope for their forgiveness in return, and to let the past go regardless of the outcome. After this they hope to be better able to listen to people, accept them, and respond to them from their deepest essence, accessible through their heart in love. There are some powerful healing principles in these steps for everyone, not just those with alcoholic addiction. Serve first, and then lead by example. Live with an open heart, even if it gets broken along the way. Be tender; be vulnerable with someone. Take emotional risks, but acknowledge and tend to your emotions.

Sacrificial Heart

Spirit is represented by a sacrificial heart. Johann Wolfgang Von Goethe (1749–1832), seventeenth-century German poet, dramatist, and novelist, said, "He who is plenteously provided for from within, needs but little from without." Consider sacrificing a weekend to go on a spiritual retreat. There you will learn more about your innermost thoughts and fears and be able to confront them. You will learn about miracles. Being involved in, and reacting to, the births and deaths of family and other significant people can provide important spiritual education. These experiences give us unexpected messages for growth and teach us about God. We oftentimes can reflect more deeply and personally on these life passages during our quiet times in spiritual retreats. It is healthy to process times of transition and ultimately relate them to our own life transitions. God is the conductor of a symphony, and we are the musicians playing the instruments. If we all pay close attention to the conductor, the universe often returns to us peace, order, and valuable information for health and soul healing. Spiritual retreats provide excellent venues for silence and reflection to allow deep, unresolved conflicts to surface and be recognized and addressed. I highly recommend you consider not just one retreat but several, for renewal and refreshment along your health journey.

Generous Heart

The last aspect of spiritual self involves our social health represented by a generous heart. We were created to serve and to be community minded. Every situation, challenge, and relationship contains some lesson worth teaching to or sharing with others. Volunteer, give your time and talents, and get involved in your community.

Empowerment, Accountability, and Belief

Chuck Swindoll, a Christian pastor, author, and radio host, writes, "The most significant decision I make each day is my choice of an attitude. When my attitudes are right, there's no barrier too high, no valley too deep, no dream too extreme, no challenge too great for me." Believe in the elegance of simple living. Herbert Benson, MD, professor of medicine at Harvard, states, "I am astonished that my studies have so conclusively shown that our bodies are wired to believe. Believe in something good if you can. Or even better, believe in something better than anything you can fathom." Read the Bible and other divinely inspired literature. William Mather Lewis tells us that abundant life does not come to those who have had a lot of obstacles removed from their paths by others. It develops from within and is rooted in strong mental and moral fiber. It is enlightened and accountable.

I will close with an exercise in guided imagery. Have you heard of *The Creation*, by Franz Joseph Haydn? It's a magnificent oratorio. The lyrics are based on Milton's *Paradise Lost*. There were three angels who were allowed to come down from heaven and witness God's creation—Raphael, Gabriel, and Uriel. Right now, pretend you are Raphael. This is day two after dry land and water were created, and, as Raphael, you will watch as the mountains and oceans are created. Try to visualize this scene. Better yet, rent the CD and listen to the music, or read the lyrics and meditate on the scene. Hear how the orchestra paints the lyrics on your heart.

> Rolling in foaming billows
> Tumultuous roars the boisterous sea.
> Mountains and rocks now emerge.
> Their tops into the clouds ascend.

> Through the open plains outstretching wide
> Full flows the gathering stream and winding wanders
> Softly purling glides on
> Through silent glades the crystal brook.

And God saw that it was good. The Creation is about love. Love is life's most precious gift of all. May you be blessed with the simple abundance of love in your journey toward holistic healing.

> *Adopt the pace of nature; her secret is patience.*
> —RALPH WALDO EMERSON

About the Author

Dr. Cathy Rosenbaum is a holistic clinical pharmacist, certified health coach, and the founder and CEO of a consulting practice in holistic health, Rx Integrative Solutions. She believes that prescription drugs and dietary supplements are running our lives and that there is a more sustainable path to wellness. The path starts with back-to-basics living and the Eight-Balance-Point Model for Healing.

Dr. Rosenbaum received her BS in pharmacy from Ohio Northern University, her PharmD from the University of Cincinnati, and her MBA from Xavier University. She is a member of the Academy of Integrative Health and Medicine, the American Society of Health Systems Pharmacists, American College of Healthcare Executives, and the Association of Natural Medicine Pharmacists. She is also a member of the Cancer Support Center Professional Advisory Board in Blue Ash, Ohio, and the professional editorial boards for *Pharmacy Practice News* and *Holistic Primary Care*. She has authored multiple peer-reviewed publications in medical literature.

Dr. Rosenbaum has a background in the pharmaceutical industry, hospital-based pharmacy practice, academia, medication quality and safety, and integrative health and medicine consulting. In 2002 she traveled to China to study herbal research and global healthcare solutions.

Over the past fifteen years, Dr. Rosenbaum has consulted with clients in partnership with their doctors to review drug and supplement interactions, side effects, product quality, and cost and to minimize the number of products whenever possible.

Dr. Rosenbaum hosts a talk-radio show called *Your Holistic Health*, a wellness program that gives listeners practical tips on how to integrate body, mind, and spiritual principles into everyday living. She has been interviewed on multiple radio and TV shows around the United States. For more information, visit www.rxintegrativesolutions.com.

APPENDIX

References for Chapter 3—The Prescription-Drug Industry

Asztalos B. F., M. Batista, K. V. Horvath, C. E. Cox, G. E. Dallal, J. S. Morse, G. B. Brown, and E. J Schaefer. 2003. "Change in Alpha1 HDL Concentration Predicts Progression in Coronary Artery Stenosis." *Arter Thromb Vasc Biol* 23: 847–852.

Bailey, R. L., J. J. Galiche, P. E. Miller, P. R. Thomas, and J. T. Dwyer. 2013. "Why US Adults Use Dietary Supplements." *JAMA Intern Med* 173: 335–361.

Cole, M. R., and C. W. Fetrow. 2003. "Adulteration of Dietary Supplements. *Am J Health Syst Pharm* 60: 1576–1580.

Dormann, H., M. Criegee-Rieck, and A. Neubert. 2003. "Lack of Awareness of Community-Acquired Adverse Drug Reactions upon Hospital Admission: Dimensions and Consequences of a Dilemma." *Drug Safety* 26: 353–362.

Gardiner, P., R. E. Graham, A. T. Legedza, D. M. Eisenberg, and R. S. Phillips. 2006. "Factors Associated with Dietary Supplement Use among Prescription Medication Users." *Arch Intern Med* 166: 1968–1974.

IMS Institute for Healthcare Informatics. April 2012. "The Use of Medicines in the United States: Review of 2011." http://www.imshealth.com/ims/Global/Content/Insights/IMS%20Institute%20for%20Healthcare%20Informatics/IHII_Medicines_in_U.S_Report_2011.pdf.

Kripke, D. F., R. D. Langer, and L. E. Kline. 2012. "Hypnotics' Association with Mortality or Cancer: a Matched Cohort Study." *BMJ Open* February 27. doi: 10.1136/bmjopen-2012-000850.

Lasser K. E., P. D. Allen, S. J. Woolhandler, S. M. Wolfe, D. H. Bor. 2002. "Timing of New Black-Box Warnings and Withdrawals for Prescription Medications." *JAMA* 287: 2215–2220.

Lazarou J., B. H. Pomeranz, and P. N. Corey. 1998. "Incidence of adverse drug reactions in hospitalized patients: A meta-analysis of prospective studies." *JAMA* 279: 1200–1205.

Qato, D. M., G. C. Alexander, R. M. Conti, M. Johnson, P. Schumm, and S. T. Lindau. 2008. "Use of Prescription and Over-the-Counter Medications and Dietary Supplements among Older Adults in the United States." *JAMA* 300 (2): 2867–2878.

Reinhart K. M., and J. A. Woods. 2012. "Strategies to Preserve the Use of Statins in Patients with Previous Muscular Adverse Effects." *Am J Health Syst Pharm* 69: 291–300.

References for Chapter 4—Herbs, Other Dietary Supplements, and Nutrition

Anon. 1984. "Toxic Effects of Vitamin Overdosage." *Medical Letter on Drugs and Therapeutics* 26: 73–4.

Braun L. A., E. Tiralongo, J. M. Wilkinson, O. Spitzer, M. Bailey, S. Poole, and M. Doole. 2010. "Perceptions, Use and Attitudes of Pharmacy Customers on Complementary Medicines and Pharamcy Practice." *BMC Complement Altern Med* 10: 38.

Buettner, C., K. J. Mukamal, P. Gardiner, R. B. Davis, R. S. Phillips, and M. A. Mittleman. 2009. "Herbal Supplement Use and Blood Lead Levels of United States Adults." *J Gen Intern Med* 24: 1175–1182.

Cohen, P. A. "American Roulette—Contaminated Dietary Supplements." *N Engl J Med* October 8, 2009. doi: 10.1056/NEHNp0904768.

Eisenberg, D. M., R. C. Kessler, C. Foster, F. E. Norlock, D. R. Calkins, and T. L. Delbanco. 1993. "Unconventional Medicine in the United States. Prevalence, Costs, and Patterns of Use." *N Engl J Med* 328: 246–252.

Ekor, M. 2014. "The Growing Use of Herbal Medicines: Issues Relating to Adverse Reactions and Challenges in Monitoring Safety." *Frontiers in Pharmacology* 4: 1–10.

Fugh-Berman, A. 2000. "Herb-Drug Interactions." *Lancet* 355: 134–138.

Gardiner, P., R. Graham, A. T. Legedza, A. C. Ahn, D. M. Eisenberg, and R. S. Phillips. 2007. "Factors Associated with Herbal Therapy Use by Adults in the United States." *Altern Ther Health Med* 13: 22–29.

Gurley, B. J. 2009. "Clinical Pharmacology and Dietary Supplements: an Evolving Relationship." *Clin Pharmacology Therapeutics*, November 25, 2009. doi: 10.1038/clpt.:245.

Matanovic, M. S., and V. Vlahovic-Palcevski. 2012. "Potentially Inappropriate Medications in the Elderly: a Comprehensive Protocol." *Eur J Clin Pharmacol* Feb 24 PMID 22362342.

Navarro, V. J. 2009. "Herbal and Dietary Supplement Hepatotoxicity." *Sem Liver Disease* 29: 373–382.

Ramanathan, V. S., G. Hensley, S. French, V. Eysselein, D. Chung, S. Reicher, and B. Pham. 2009. "Hypervitaminosis A Inducing Intra-Hepatic Cholestasis—a Rare Case Report. *Experimental Molecular Pathology*. doi: 10.1016/j.yexmp.2009.11.007.

Saper, R. B., R. S. Phillips, A. Schgal, N. Khouri, R. B. David, J. Paquin, V. Thuppil, and S. N. Kales. 2008. "Lead, Mercury, and Arsenic in US- and Indian-Manufactured Ayurvedic Medicines Sold via the Internet. *JAMA* 300 (8): 915–923.

Shaw, D., G. Ladds, P. Duez, E. Williamson, and K. Chan. 2012. "Pharmacovigilance of Herbal Medicine." *J Ethnopharmacology* doi: 10/1016/j.jep.2012.01.051.

Stanger, M. J., L. A. Thompson, A. J. Young, and H. R. Lieberman. 2012. "Anticoagulant Activity of Select Dietary Supplements." *Nutrition Reviews* 70: 107–117.

Verkaik-Kloosterman J., M. T. McCann, J. Hoekstra, and H. Verhagen. 2012. "Vitamins and Minerals: Issues Assocaied with Too Low and Too High Population Intakes." *Food & Nutrition Research* 56: 5728–5732.

References for Chapter 5—Complementary and Alternative Medicine
Balneaves, L. G., T. Truant, M. Verhoef, B. Ross, A. Porcino, M. Wong, and A. S. Brazier. 2010. "The Complementary Medicine Education and Outcomes (CAMEO) Program: a Foundation for Patient and Health Professional Education and Decision Support Programs." *Patient Educ Couns* doi: 10.1016/j.pec.201.01.005.

Benjamin, R. National Prevention, Health Promotions, and Public Health Council. 2013. "Annual Status Report" http://www.surgeongeneral.gov/initiatives/prevention/2013-npc-status-report.pdf accessed on 6/29/15.

Colloca, Luana, and D. Finniss. 2012. "Nocebo Effects, Patient-Clinician Communication, and Therapeutic Outcomes." *JAMA* 307: 567–568.

Kaptchuk, T. J., J. Shaw, C. E. Kerr, L. A. Conboy, J. M. Kelley, and T. J. Csordas. 2009. "'Maybe I Made up the Whole Thing': Placebos and Patients' Experiences in a Randomized Controlled Trial." *Cult Med Psychiatry* 33: 382–411. doi: 10.1007/s11013-009-9141-7.

Kessler, R. C., R. B. Davis, and D. F. Foster. 2001. "Long Term Trends in the Use of Complementary and Alternative Medical Therapies in the United States." *Ann Intern Med* 135: 262–8.

Miller, F. G., E. J. Emanuel, D. L. Rosenstein, S. E. Straus. 2004." Ethical Issues Concerning Research in Complementary and Alternative Medicine." *JAMA* 291: 599–604.

O'Connell, N. E., B. M. Wand, and B. Goldacre. 2009. "Interpretive Bias in Acupuncture Research? A Case Study." *Eval and Health Professions* 32: 393–409.

Park, A. "America's Health Checkup." *Time*. November 20, 2008.

Pilkington, K., and A. Boshnakova. 2012. "Complementary Medicine and Safety: a Systematic Investigation of Design and Reporting of Systematic Reviews." *Complementary Therapies in Medicine* 20: 73–82.

References for Chapter 6—Personalized Health and Wellness

Briggs Myers, I., P. B. Myers. 1995. *Gifts Differing: Understanding Personality Type*. Mountain View, CA: Davies-Black Publishing.

Brown, J. 2011. "Laughter as Medicine." *CDS Rev* 104: 26–27.

Caire-Juvera, G., C. Ritenbaugh, J. Wactawski-Wende, L. G. Snetselaar, and Z. Chen. 2009. "Vitamin A and Retinol Intakes and the Risk of Fractures among Participants of the Women's Health Initiative Observational Study." *Am J Clin Nutr* 89: 323–330.

Gaudia, G. 2007. "About Intercessory Prayer: the Scientific Study of Miracles." *Med Gen Med* 9(1): 55–56.

Goleman, D. 1998. *Working with Emotional Intelligence*. New York, NY: Bantam Books.

Greenleaf, R. 2002. *Servant Leadership*. Paulist Press. New York.

Jonas, W. B. 2001. "The Middle Way: Realistic Randomized Controlled Trials for the Evaluation of Spiritual Healing." *J Comp Alt Med* 7: 5–7.

Kris-Etherton, P., R. H. Eckel, V. V. Howard, S. St Jeor, and T. L. Bazzarre. 2001. Nutrition Committee Population Science Committee and Clinical Science Committee of the American Heart Association. AHA Science Advisory: Lyon Diet Heart Study. *Circulation* 103: 1823–1825.

Kuchan, K. L. 2008. "Prayer as Therapeutic Process toward Aliveness within a Spiritual Direction Relationship." *J Relig Health* 47: 263–275. doi: 10.1007/s10943-007-9153-y.

Larimore, W. L., M. Parker, and M. Crowther. 2002. "Should Clinicians Incorporate Positive Spirituality in Their Practices? What Does the Evidence Say?" *Ann Behav Med* 24: 69–73.

Ludwig, D. S., and J. Kabat-Zinn. 2008. "Mindfulness in Medicine." *JAMA* 300: 1350–1352.

Norcross, J. C., P. M. Krebs, and J. O. Prochaska. 2011. "Stages of Change." *J Clin Psychol* 67: 143–154.

O'Hara, D. P. 2002. "Is There a Role for Prayer and Spirituality in Health Care?" *Med Clin North Am* 86: 33–46.

Palmer, H. 1995. *The Enneagram in Love and Work. Understanding Your Intimate and Business Relationships.* Harper Collins.

Palmer, R. F., D. Katerndahl, and J. Morgan-Kidd. 2004. "A Randomized Trial of the Effects of Remote Intercessory Prayer: Interactions with Personal Beliefs on Problem-Specific Outcomes and Functional Status." *J Altern Complement Med* 10: 438–48.

Rosenbaum, C. C. 2007. "The Role of the Pharmacist in Prayer and Spirituality." *Annals Pharmacotherapy* 41: 505–507.

Sweeney, T. J. The Wellness and Habit Change Workbook 2004.

University of Maryland Medical Center. "Spirituality." http://www.umm.edu/altmed/articles/spirituality-000360.htm how does spirituality influence health. Accessed June 27, 2015.

References for Chapter 7—Combating Superstress with Guided Imagery

Boehm, L. B., and A. M. Tse. 2013. "Application of Guided Imagery to Facilitate the Transition of New Graduate Registered Nurses." *J Contin Educ Nurs* 44(3): 113–9.

Grenny, J., R. McMillan, and A. Switzler. 2002. *Crucial Conversations: Tools for Talking When Stakes Are High*. McGraw Hill.

Holmes, T. H., and R. Rahe. 1967. "The Social Readjustment Rating Scale." *Journal of Psychosomatic Research* 11 (2): 213–218.

Menzies, V., D. E. Lyon, R. K. Elswick Jr., N. L. McCain, and D. P. Gray. 2014. "Effects of Guided Imagery on Biobehavioral Factors in Women with Fibromyalgia." *J Behav Med* 37(1): 70–80.

Mizrahi, M. C., R. Reicher-Atir, S. Levy, S. Haramati, D. Wengrower, E. Israeli, and E. Goldin. 2012. "Effects of Guided Imagery with Relaxation Training on Anxiety and Quality of Life among Patients with Inflammatory Bowel Disease." *Psychol Health* 27(12): 1463–79.

Schaffer, L, N. Jallo, L. Howland, K. James, D. Glaser, and K. Arnell. 2013. "Guided Imagery: an Innovative Approach to Improving Maternal Sleep Quality." *J Perinat Neonatal Nurs* 27(2): 151–9.

References for Chapter 8—Aromatherapy

Bent, S. 2000. "Aromatherapy: Ineffective Treatment or Effective Placebo?" *Eff Clin Pract* 4: 188–190.

Cooke, B., and E. Ernst. 2000. "Aromatherapy: a Systematic Review." *Br J Gen Pract* 50: 493–496.

Fismer, K. L., and K. Pilkington. 2012. "Lavender and Sleep: a Systematic Review of the Evidence." *Euro J Integrative Med* 4(4): e436–e447. doi: 10.1016/j.eujim.2012.08.001.

Hunt, R., J. Dienermann, H. J. Norton, W. Hartley, A. Hudgens, T. Stern, and G. Divine. 2013. "Aromatherapy as Treatment for Postoperative Nausea: a Randomized Trial." *Anesth Analg* 117(3): 597–604. doi: 10.1213/ANE.0b013e31824a0b1c.

Papadopoulos, A., S. Wright, and J. Ensor. 1999. "Evaluation and Attributional Analysis of an Aromatherapy Service for Older Adults with Physical Health Problems and Carers Using the Service." *Compl Ther Med* 7: 239–244.

Saeki, Y. 2000. "The Effect of Foot-Bath with or without the Essential Oil of Lavender on the Autonomic Nervous System: a Randomized Trial." *Compl Ther Med* 8: 2–7.

Sarris, J. 2001. "A Systematic Review of Insomnia and Complementary Medicine." *Sleep Med Rev* 15: 99–106.

Sayorwan, W., N. Ruangrungsi, T. Piriyapunyporn, T. Hongratanaworakit, N. Kotchabhakdi, and V. Siripornpanich. 2013. "Effects of Inhaled Rosemary Oil on Subjective Feelings and Activities of the Nervous System." *Sci Pharm* 81(2): 531–542. doi: 10.3797/scipharm.1209-05.

Sayorwan, W., V. Siripornpanich, T. Piriyapunyaporn, T. Hongratanaworakit, N. Kotchabhakdi, and N. Ruangrungsi. 2012. "The Effects of Lavender Oil Inhalation on Emotional States, Autonomic Nervous System, and Brain Electrical Activity." *J Med Assoc Thai* 95(4): 598–606.

Setzer, W. 2009. "Essential Oils and Anxiolytic Aromatherapy." *Nat Prod Commun* 4: 1305–1306.

Soo Lee, M., J. Choi, P. Posadzki, and E. Ernst. 2012. "Aromatherapy for Health Care: an Overview of Systematic Reviews." *Maturitas* 71: 257–260.

References for Chapter 9—Spiritual Renewal

Fraley H., E. J. Theissen, and S. Jiwanlal. 2014. "Spiritual Care in a Crisis: What is Enough?" *Christ Nurs* 31: 161–165.

Hills, J., J. A. Paice, J. R. Cameron, and S. Shott. 2005. "Spirituality and Distress in Palliative Care Consultation." *J Palliative Med* 8: 782–788.

Kuczewski, M. G. 2007. "Talking about Spirituality in the Clinical Setting: Can Being Professional Require Being Personal?" *Am J Bioeth* 7: 4–11.

Ledger, S. D. 2005. "The Duty of Nurses to Meet Patients' Spiritual and /or Religious Needs." *Br J Nursing* 14: 220–225.

Lorenz, F. O., R. D. Conger, and G. H. Elder. 2006. "The Short-Term and Decade-Long Effects of Divorce on Women's Midlife Health." *J Health Social Behavior* 47: 111–125.

McKnight, C. M., and S. Juillerat. 2001. "Perceptions of Clinical Athletic Trainers on the Spiritual Care of Injured Athletes. *J Athl Train* 46(3): 303–311.

Ng, S. M., J. K. Y. Yu, C. L. W. Chan, C. H. Y. Chan, and D. Y. F. Ho. 2005. "The Measurement of Body-Mind-Spirit Well-Being: Toward Multidimensionality and Transcultural Applicability." *Social Work in Health Care* 41: 33–52.

Oman, D., and J. Hedberg. 2006. "Passage Meditation Reduces Perceived Stress in Health Professionals: a Randomized, Controlled Trial." *J Consulting Clin Psychology* 74: 714–719.

Phillips, L. L., A. L. Paukert, M. A. Stanley, and M. E. Kunik. 2009. "Incorporating Religion and Spirituality to Improve Care for Anxiety and Depression in Older Adults." *Geriatrics* 64: 15–8.

Struve, J. K. 2002. "Faith's Impact on Health. Implications for the Practice of Medicine. *Minn Med* 85(12): 41–44.

Tuck, I., R. Alleyne, and W. Thinganjana. 2006. "Spirituality and Stress Management in Healthy Adults." *J Holistic Nursing* 24: 245–253.

Thornton, L. 2005. "The Model of Whole Person Caring." *Holistic Nurs Pract* 19: 106–115.

Williams, L., R. Gorman, and S. Hankerson. 2014. "Implementing a Mental Health Ministry Committee in Faith-Based Organizations: the Promoting Emotional Wellness and Spirituality Program." *Soc Work Health Care* 53(4): 414–434.

INDEX

Index	Page
Academy for Guided Imagery	39, 60
Acupuncture	37, 39
Addiction	17
Affordable Care Act	4
Alcoholics Anonymous	66
American Academy of Medical Acupuncture	39
American Botanical Council	29
American Herbalists Guild	29
American Massage Therapy Association	39
American Meditation Institute	39
American Music Therapy Association	39
Anti-inflammatory	47
Antioxidants	47
Aromatherapy	28, 37, 39, 61
Association for Applied and Therapeutic Humor	39
Association of Natural Medicine Pharmacists	39
Baby Boomers	4
Bee Balm	49
Bible	6, 65, 67
British Herbal Medicine Association	29
Cardamom Essential Oil	63
Chamomile	49
China	11-13
Chuck Swindoll	67
Cinnamon Essential Oil	62
Clinical Trials	17, 18
College of Practitioners of Phytotherapy	29
Complementary and Alternative Medicine	36-41, 43, 44, 46, 50, 55, 60
Consumer Labs	33
Decoctions	28, 29

Dietary Supplement	15, 22, 23, 25, 27-37, 39, 43, 46
Dietary Supplement Health and Education Act	31, 32
Dill Essential Oil	63
DISC Assessment	50
Drug Adulteration	25
Drug Interactions	21, 25, 34
Drug Shortages	18-21
Eight-Balance-Point Model for Healing	41, 43, 45, 55
Emotional Health	50
Enneagram	50
Environmental Health	52
Ephedra Sinica	34
Essential Oils	28, 30, 61-63
Eucalyptus Essential Oil	63
European Scientific Cooperative on Phytotherapy	30
Exercise	48
Extracts	28, 29
FDA	11, 14, 16-19, 21, 23-25, 30, 32, 33
Forgiveness	53, 66
Frankincense Essential Oil	63
German Commission E Monographs	30
Ginger	35, 63
Ginkgo Biloba	34
Good Manufacturing Practice	18-20
Grapefruit (*Citrus paradisi*) Essential Oil	63
Green Tea	49
Guided Imagery	39, 56, 59, 60, 67
Herbs	28-30, 32-35
Holistic	37, 60, 68
Holmes and Rahe Stress Scale	56, 57
Infusions	29
Institute of Medicine	31
Integrative Health and Medicine	37
Jasmine Essential Oil	63

Jonquil Essential Oil	63
Kava Kava	35
Laughter Therapy	39, 51
Lavender	49, 61, 63
Lemon Essential Oil	62, 63
Licorice	34, 35
Life Purpose	54
Lime Essential Oil	62, 63
Livestrong Foundation	25
Mandarin Essential Oil	63
Massage	37, 39, 62, 65
Mayo Clinic	25
Mediterranean Diet	28, 46
Meditation	63
Menopause	14, 15, 35
Mind-Body Connection	57
Miracles	7-10
Myers Briggs Personality Test	50
National Association for Holistic Aromatherapy	39
National Center for Complementary and Integrative Health	33
National Institute of Medical Herbalists	29
Nocebo Effect	40
Nutrition	46-48
Orange (*Citrus sinensis*) Essential Oil	63
Oregano	62
People's Pharmacy	25
Peppermint Essential Oil	63
PhRMA	16, 21
Physical Health	45, 46
Placebo Effect	40
Polypharmacy	21, 46
Prayer	53
Prescription Medications	14-25
Pubmed.gov	25
Readiness for Change	44, 45

Relationship Health	51
Rose Essential Oil	63
Rosewood Essential Oil	63
Sandalwood Essential Oil	63
Servant Leadership	54, 66
SFDA	11, 12
Sleep	49, 63
Spearmint Essential Oil	63
Spiritual Health	39, 52, 53, 64-67
Superstress	56-59
Sweet Orange Essential Oil	62
US Pharmacopoeia	31
The Blue Zones	54
The Creation	67, 68
Thyme	62
Tinctures	28, 29
Traditional Chinese Medicine	11
Vitamins	48
Worship	54
Zumba	38, 48

NOTES

NOTES

NOTES

NOTES

NOTES